Updates in Obstetric and Gynecologic Emergencies

Editors

BRITTANY GUEST
SARAH B. DUBBS

EMERGENCY MEDICINE
CLINICS OF NORTH AMERICA

www.emed.theclinics.com

Consulting Editor
AMAL MATTU

May 2023 • Volume 41 • Number 2

ELSEVIER

1600 John F. Kennedy Boulevard • Suite 1800 • Philadelphia, Pennsylvania, 19103-2899

http://www.theclinics.com

EMERGENCY MEDICINE CLINICS OF NORTH AMERICA Volume 41, Number 2
May 2023 ISSN 0733-8627, ISBN-13: 978-0-323-93951-5

Editor: Joanna Gascoine
Developmental Editor: Axell Ivan Jade Purificacion

© **2023 Elsevier Inc. All rights reserved.**

This periodical and the individual contributions contained in it are protected under copyright by Elsevier, and the following terms and conditions apply to their use:

Photocopying
Single photocopies of single articles may be made for personal use as allowed by national copyright laws. Permission of the Publisher and payment of a fee is required for all other photocopying, including multiple or systematic copying, copying for advertising or promotional purposes, resale, and all forms of document delivery. Special rates are available for educational institutions that wish to make photocopies for non-profit educational classroom use. For information on how to seek permission visit www.elsevier.com/permissions or call: (+44) 1865 843830 (UK)/(+1) 215 239 3804 (USA).

Derivative Works
Subscribers may reproduce tables of contents or prepare lists of articles including abstracts for internal circulation within their institutions. Permission of the Publisher is required for resale or distribution outside the institution. Permission of the Publisher is required for all other derivative works, including compilations and translations (please consult www.elsevier.com/permissions).

Electronic Storage or Usage
Permission of the Publisher is required to store or use electronically any material contained in this periodical, including any article or part of an article (please consult www.elsevier.com/permissions). Except as outlined above, no part of this publication may be reproduced, stored in a retrieval system or transmitted in any form or by any means, electronic, mechanical, photocopying, recording or otherwise, without prior written permission of the Publisher.

Notice
No responsibility is assumed by the Publisher for any injury and/or damage to persons or property as a matter of products liability, negligence or otherwise, or from any use or operation of any methods, products, instructions or ideas contained in the material herein. Because of rapid advances in the medical sciences, in particular, independent verification of diagnoses and drug dosages should be made.

Although all advertising material is expected to conform to ethical (medical) standards, inclusion in this publication does not constitute a guarantee or endorsement of the quality or value of such product or of the claims made of it by its manufacturer.

Emergency Medicine Clinics of North America (ISSN 0733-8627) is published quarterly by Elsevier Inc., 360 Park Avenue South, New York, NY, 10010-1710. Months of issue are February, May, August, and November. Business and Editorial Offices: 1600 John F. Kennedy Boulevard, Suite 1800, Philadelphia, PA 19103-2899. Customer Service Office: 6277 Sea Harbor Drive, Orlando, FL 32887-4800. Periodicals postage paid at New York, NY, and additional mailing offices. Subscription prices are $100.00 per year (US students), $381.00 per year (US individuals), $778.00 per year (US institutions), $220.00 per year (international students), $490.00 per year (international individuals), $958.00 per year (international institutions), $100.00 per year (Canadian students), $449.00 per year (Canadian individuals), and $958.00 per year (Canadian institutions). International air speed delivery is included in all *Clinics'* subscription prices. All prices are subject to change without notice. **POSTMASTER:** Send address changes to *Emergency Medicine Clinics of North America*, Elsevier Periodicals Customer Service, 11830 Westline Industrial Drive, St. Louis, MO 63146. Customer Service (orders, claims, online, change of address): Elsevier Periodicals **Customer Service, 11830 Westline Industrial Drive, St. Louis, MO 63146. Tel: 1-800-654-2452 (U.S. and Canada); 314-453-7041 (outside U.S. and Canada). Fax: 314-453-5170. E-mail: journalscustomerservice-usa@elsevier.com (for print support); journalsonlinesupport-usa@elsevier.com (for online support).**

Reprints. For copies of 100 or more of articles in this publication, please contact the Commercial Reprints Department, Elsevier Inc., 360 Park Avenue South, New York, NY 10010-1710. Tel.: 212-633-3874; Fax: 212-633-3820; E-mail: reprints@elsevier.com.

Emergency Medicine Clinics of North America is covered in *MEDLINE/PubMed (Index Medicus), Current Contents/Clinical Medicine, EMBASE/Excerpta Medica, BIOSIS, SciSearch, CINAHL, ISI/BIOMED,* and *Research Alert.*

Contributors

CONSULTING EDITOR

AMAL MATTU, MD
Professor and Vice Chair of Academic Affairs, Department of Emergency Medicine, University of Maryland School of Medicine, Baltimore, Maryland

EDITORS

BRITTANY GUEST, DO
Assistant Clinical Professor, Department of Emergency Medicine, David Geffen School of Medicine at UCLA, Director of EM:RAPs Live and Virtual Events, Los Angeles, California

SARAH B. DUBBS, MD
Associate Professor, Department of Emergency Medicine, University of Maryland School of Medicine, Baltimore, Maryland

AUTHORS

REBECCA A. BAVOLEK, MD, FACEP, FAAEM
Clinical Professor of Emergency Medicine, Vice Chair of Education, Residency Program Director, UCLA-Ronald Reagan/Olive View Emergency Medicine Residency, Los Angeles, California

MICHELE CALLAHAN, MD
Adjunct Assistant Professor, Department of Emergency Medicine, University of Maryland School of Medicine, Baltimore, Maryland USA

BENJAMIN CHAN, MD, MPH
UCLA Ronald Reagan | Olive View, Los Angeles, California

CALEB CHAN, MD
Assistant Professor, Department of Medicine, University of Maryland Medical Center, Department of Emergency Medicine, University of Maryland School of Medicine, Baltimore, Maryland

NICOLE CIMINO-FIALLOS, MD, FACEP, FAAEM
Assistant Medical Director, Emergency Department, Meritus Health, US Acute Care Solutions, Hagerstown, Maryland

NATHANIEL COGGINS, MD
UCLA-Ronald Reagan/Olive View Emergency Medicine Program, Los Angeles, California

JESSICA DOWNING, MD
Surgical Critical Care Fellow, R Adams Cowley Shock Trauma Center, University of Maryland Medical Center, Baltimore, Maryland

PAMELA L. DYNE, MD, FACEP
Chief Physician Wellbeing Officer, Olive View-UCLA Medical Center, Professor of Clinical Emergency Medicine, UCLA David Geffen School of Medicine, Sylmar, California

KAMI M. HU, MD, FAAEM, FACEP
Department of Emergency Medicine, Department of Internal Medicine, Division of Pulmonary & Critical Care, University of Maryland School of Medicine, Baltimore Maryland, USA

SAMANTHA A. KING, MD
Assistant Professor, Department of Emergency Medicine, University of Maryland School of Medicine, Baltimore, Maryland

KELLIE KITAMURA, MD
Assistant Clinical Professor and Associate Program Director, UCLA-Ronald Reagan/Olive View Emergency Medicine Program, Los Angeles, California

DIANE KUHN, MD, PhD
Assistant Professor of Clinical Emergency Medicine, Department of Emergency Medicine, Indiana University School of Medicine, Indianapolis, Indiana

STEVEN LAI, MD
UCLA-Ronald Reagan/Olive View Emergency Medicine Program, Assistant Clinical Professor and Associate Program Director, Los Angeles, California

VIVIAN LAM, MD, MPH
Department of Internal Medicine, Section of Critical Care Medicine, Advocate Christ Medical Center, Oak Lawn, Illinois

SARA MANNING, MD
Assistant Professor of Emergency Medicine, Assistant Clerkship Director, Department of Emergency Medicine, Indiana University School of Medicine, Indianapolis, Indiana

NASEEM MORIDZADEH, MD
Clinical Instructor, NYU Langone Health, Los Angeles, California

CAITLIN L. OLDENKAMP, MD
Chief Resident Physician, UCLA-Ronald Reagan/Olive View Emergency Medicine Program, Los Angeles, California

BENITO NIKOLAS PASCUA, MD
UCLA Emergency Medicine, Los Angeles, California

EMILY ROSE, MD
Associate Professor of Clinical Emergency Medicine (Educational Scholar), Director, Pre-Health Undergraduate Studies, Department of Emergency Medicine, Keck School of Medicine of the University of Southern California, Los Angeles County + University of Southern California Medical Center, Old General Hospital, Los Angeles, California

CAROLYN JOY SACHS, MD, MPH
UCLA Ronald Reagan | Olive View, Los Angeles, California

ALEXIS SALERNO, MD, AEMUS-FPD
Assistant Professor, Department of Emergency Medicine, University of Maryland School of Medicine, Advanced Emergency Medicine Ultrasonography Fellowship Director, Baltimore, Maryland

JOHN MARK SAWYER, MD
Resident Physician, UCLA-Ronald Reagan/Olive View Emergency Medicine Residency, Los Angeles, California

LUCAS SJEKLOCHA, MD
Assistant Professor, Department of Emergency Medicine, Program in Trauma, R Adams Cowley Shock Trauma Center, University of Maryland School of Medicine, Baltimore, Maryland

CHEYENNE SNAVELY, MD
Critical Care Fellow, Department of Medicine, University of Maryland Medical Center, Baltimore, Maryland

SARAH SOMMERKAMP, MD
Assistant Professor, Department of Emergency Medicine, University of Maryland School of Medicine, Baltimore, Maryland

MARISSA WOLFE, MD
Chief Resident, Los Angeles County + University of Southern California Medical Center, Los Angeles, California

Contributors

ALEXIS SALERNO, MD, AEMUS-FPD
Assistant Professor, Department of Emergency Medicine, University of Maryland School of Medicine, Advanced Emergency Medicine Ultrasonography Fellowship Director, Baltimore, Maryland

JOHN MARK SAWYER, MD
Research Physician, UCLA Ronald Reagan/Olive View Emergency Medicine Residency, Los Angeles, California

LUCAS SJEKLOCHA, MD
Assistant Professor, Department of Emergency Medicine, Program in Trauma, R Adams Cowley Shock Trauma Center, University of Maryland School of Medicine, Baltimore, Maryland

CHEYENNE SHAVELL, MD
Critical Care Fellow, Department of Medicine, University of Maryland Medical Center, Baltimore, Maryland

SARAH SOMMERKAMP, MD
Associate Professor, Department of Emergency Medicine, University of Maryland School of Medicine, Baltimore, Maryland

MARISSA WOLFE, MD
Chief Resident, Los Angeles County/University of Southern California Medical Center, Los Angeles, California

Contents

Foreword: Updates in Obstetric and Gynecologic Emergencies　　　　　　xiii

Amal Mattu

Preface: The Emergency Department Safety Net for Obstetric/Gynecologic Emergencies　　　　　　xv

Brittany Guest and Sarah B. Dubbs

Trauma in Pregnancy　　　　　　223

Jessica Downing and Lucas Sjeklocha

Trauma is the leading cause of nonobstetric maternal death. Pregnant patients have a similar spectrum of traumatic injuries with a noted increase in interpersonal violence. A structured approach to trauma evaluation and management is recommended with several guidelines expanding on advanced trauma life support (ATLS) principles; however, evidence is limited. Optimal management requires understanding of physiologic changes in pregnancy, a team-based approach, and preparation for interventions that may including neonatal resuscitation. The principles of trauma management are the same in pregnancy with a systematic approach and initial maternal focused resuscitation.

Cardiovascular Complications of Pregnancy　　　　　　247

John Mark Sawyer, Naseem Moridzadeh, and Rebecca A. Bavolek

The physiologic changes in pregnancy predispose the pregnant patient to a variety of potential cardiovascular complications. In this article, we discuss the major cardiovascular disorders of pregnancy and their management, highlight specific diagnostic challenges, and discuss new developments in the field. Topics covered in this article include venous thromboembolism, acute myocardial infarction, peripartum cardiomyopathy, and aortic dissection.

Nonobstetric Surgical Emergencies in Pregnancy　　　　　　259

Caitlin L. Oldenkamp and Kellie Kitamura

In this article, we discuss the major nonobstetric surgical complications that may occur in pregnancy. We highlight specific diagnostic challenges particularly with imaging modalities and radiation considerations for the fetus. Topics covered in this article include appendicitis, intestinal obstruction, gallstone disease, hepatic rupture, perforated peptic ulcer, mesenteric venous thrombosis, splenic artery aneurysm rupture, and aortic dissection.

Hypertensive Disorders of Pregnancy   269

Nathaniel Coggins and Steven Lai

> Hypertensive disorders in pregnancy are a leading cause of global maternal and fetal morbidity. The four hypertensive disorders of pregnancy include chronic hypertension, gestational hypertension, preeclampsia-eclampsia, and chronic hypertension with superimposed preeclampsia. A careful history, review of systems, physical examination, and laboratory analysis can help differentiate these disorders and quantify the severity of the disease, which holds important implications for disease management. This article reviews the different types of disorders of hypertension in pregnancy and how to diagnose and manage these patients, with special attention paid to any recent changes made to this management algorithm.

Emergency Delivery   281

Michele Callahan

> Despite the majority of US births occurring in hospitals and under the direct care of obstetricians, there is a subset of patients who will deliver imminently in the emergency department (ED). ED physicians must be skillfully trained to manage both uncomplicated and complicated delivery scenarios. An ED delivery may require resuscitation of both mother and infant, so supplies should be readily available and all necessary consultants and support staff should be involved to ensure the best outcome. Most births are uncomplicated and require no significant additional interventions but ED staff must be prepared for these more complicated scenarios.

Spontaneous and Complicated Therapeutic Abortion in the Emergency Department   295

Sara Manning and Diane Kuhn

> Pregnancy-related emergency department visits are common in the United States. Although typically managed safely in the outpatient setting, patients with spontaneous abortion may also present with life-threatening hemorrhage or infection. Management strategies for spontaneous abortion are similarly wide-ranging from expectant management to emergent surgical intervention. Surgical management of complicated therapeutic abortion is similar to that of spontaneous abortion. The dramatic changes in the legal status of abortion in the United States may have significant influence on the incidence of complicated therapeutic abortion, and we encourage emergency physicians to familiarize themselves with the diagnosis and management of these conditions.

Management of Coronavirus Disease-2019 Infection in Pregnancy   307

Vivian Lam and Kami M. Hu

> Although the majority of pregnant patients who contract the SARS-CoV 2 virus will have a mild course of illness, pregnant patients with COVID-19 are more likely than their nonpregnant counterparts to develop a severe illness with an increased risk of poor maternal and fetal outcomes. Although the extent of research in this specific patient population remains limited, there are tenets of care with which physicians and other providers must be familiar to increase the chances of better outcomes for the two patients in their care.

Resuscitation of the Obstetric Patient   323

Cheyenne Snavely and Caleb Chan

Pregnancy is a time of tremendous physiologic change and vulnerability. At any point, symptoms and complications can prompt the need for emergency care, and these can range from minor to life-threatening. Emergency physicians must be prepared to treat any of these complications, in addition to rescucitating the critically ill and injured pregnant patient. To optimally care for these patients, it is paramount to be aware of the unique physiologic changes that occur during pregnancy. The focus of this review is to discuss illnesses unique to pregnancy and additional aspects of resuscitation that must be considered when caring for a critically ill pregnant patient.

Ultrasound in Pregnancy   337

Samantha A. King, Alexis Salerno, and Sarah Sommerkamp

This article reviews the use of ultrasound in pregnancy pertinent to the emergency physician. The techniques for transabdominal and transvaginal studies are detailed including approaches to gestational dating. Diagnosis of ectopic pregnancy is reviewed focusing on the potential pitfalls: reliance on beta-human chorionic gonadotropin, pseudogestational sac, interstitial pregnancy, and heterotopic pregnancy. Techniques for the identification of placental issues and presenting parts during the second and third trimesters are reviewed. Ultrasound is a safe and effective tool for the experienced emergency physician and is integral to providing high-quality care to pregnant women.

Pediatric and Adolescent Gynecologic Emergencies   355

Marissa Wolfe and Emily Rose

Pediatric gynecology encompasses a wide range of topics from the maternal estrogen impact on the neonate, to the unique pathophysiology of the lack of estrogen on prepubescent females, and the independence and sexual maturation that occurs with adolescence. This article will review the impact of normal hormonal variations in children, unique pathophysiology of certain conditions in the prepubescent period, as well as common injuries and infections of the genitourinary system in children.

Intimate Partner Violence and Sexual Violence   369

Benjamin Chan and Carolyn Joy Sachs

Intimate partner violence and sexual violence represent significant public health challenges that carry many individual and societal costs. More than 1 in 3 women (35.6%) and more than 1 in 4 men (28.5%) in the United States have experienced rape, physical violence, and/or stalking by an intimate partner in their lifetime. Clinicians play an integral role on the screening, identification, and management of these sensitive issues.

Emergency Medicine Considerations in the Transgender Patient   381

Benito Nikolas Pascua and Pamela L. Dyne

Transgender patients are at high risk for poor health outcomes and many harbor fear of healthcare settings secondary to prior discrimination, perceived sensationalism, clinician unfamiliarity, and unwanted exams. It is essential to approach transgender patients without judgement and with empathy. Asking open ended questions with explanation as to why your questions are pertinent to their specific care will help create rapport and trust. Through a basic working knowledge of terminology, types of hormone therapy, non-surgical techniques, garments, and surgical procedures typically encountered by such patients, and their respective potential side effects and complications, clinicians can provide quality care to transgender patients.

Emergency Gynecologic Considerations in the Older Woman 395

Nicole Cimino-Fiallos and Pamela L. Dyne

As women mature through menopause, they will experience normal physiologic changes that can contribute to emergency complaints specific to this patient population. Reviewing the expected physiologic changes of menopause and correlating these normal processes to the development of specific pathologic conditions offers a framework for emergency physicians and practitioners to use when evaluating older women for breast, genitourinary, and gynecologic symptoms.

EMERGENCY MEDICINE CLINICS OF NORTH AMERICA

FORTHCOMING ISSUES

August 2023
Cardiac Arrest
William J. Brady and Amandeep Singh,
Editors

November 2023
Endocrine and Metabolic Emergencies
George Willis and Bennett A. Myers,
Editors

February 2024
Psychiatric and Behavioral Emergencies
Eileen F. Baker and Catherine A. Marco,
Editors

RECENT ISSUES

February 2023
Trauma Emergencies
Christopher Hicks and Kimberly A.
Boswell, *Editors*

November 2022
Cardiovascular Emergencies
Jeremy G. Berberian and Leen Alblaihed,
Editors

August 2022
Respiratory and Airway Emergencies
Haney Mallemat and Terren Trott, *Editors*

SERIES OF RELATED INTEREST

Obstetrics & Gynecology Clinics
https://www.obgyn.theclinics.com/
Critical Care Clinics
https://www.criticalcare.theclinics.com/

THE CLINICS ARE NOW AVAILABLE ONLINE!
Access your subscription at:
www.theclinics.com

EMERGENCY MEDICINE
CLINICS OF NORTH AMERICA

FORTHCOMING ISSUES

August 2024
Cardiac Arrest
William J. Brady and Amandeep S. Singh,
Editors

November 2023
Endocrine and Metabolic Emergencies
George Willis and Semhar Z. Myers,
Editors

February 2024
Pediatric and Adolescent Emergencies
Ellen Baker and Samantha A. Viano,
Editors

RECENT ISSUES

February 2023
Trauma Emergencies
. . . . . . and . . . . ,
Editors

November 2022
Cardiovascular Emergencies
Jenny C. Walker and Semhar Z. Abraham,
Editors

August 2022
Respiratory and Airway Emergencies
Haney Mallemat and . . . . ,
Editors

SERIES OF RELATED INTEREST

Obstetrics & Gynecology Clinics
https://www.obgyn.theclinics.com

THE CLINICS ARE NOW AVAILABLE ONLINE!
Access your subscription at:
www.theclinics.com

Foreword

Updates in Obstetric and Gynecologic Emergencies

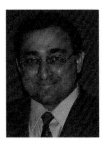

Amal Mattu, MD
Consulting Editor

If you were to ask a group of emergency physicians about which emergency department (ED) procedures produce the most stress, you'd probably hear "childbirth" as one of the most common answers. The irony here, of course, is that childbirth is not a "procedure." It is a natural process that has been occurring for thousands of years…usually with great success and without physician assistance. However, the fact that complications *sometimes* arise in this natural process, which is supposed to be associated with a happy outcome, is a major reason for the stress. The outcome of childbirth is expected by most people to be perfect, and so anything less is often blamed on the physician. Childbirth in the ED is especially complicated because it tends to occur without much advance warning in an already chaotic environment. And when things go wrong, two lives are in peril—that of an otherwise healthy young woman and that of a child. I'm getting stressed just writing about this!

Even outside of childbirth, pregnancy confers risk to two patients simultaneously when the patient presents to the ED. We in the ED are quite comfortable caring for trauma patients, cardiac patients, those with abdominal pain, and so on. But as soon as you discover that the patient is pregnant, the stress level and the risk increase significantly.

In this issue of *Emergency Medicine Clinics of North America*, Guest Editors Drs Sarah Dubbs and Brittany Guest have assembled an outstanding group of authors to assuage our feelings of stress in caring for pregnant patients. They address a multitude of patient presentations associated with pregnancy, including trauma, cardiovascular disasters, abdominal pain, hypertension, vaginal bleeding, COVID-19 infection, and emergency childbirth. Additional articles address the special issues involved in medical resuscitation as well as ultrasound. In addition to addressing obstetric issues, the contributors have also addressed several additional key topics in women's health,

Emerg Med Clin N Am 41 (2023) xiii–xiv
https://doi.org/10.1016/j.emc.2023.02.002
0733-8627/23/© 2023 Published by Elsevier Inc.

including gynecologic issues at extremes of age, transgender considerations, and intimate partner violence.

This issue of *Emergency Medicine Clinics of North America* represents an important addition to our emergency medicine libraries. Drs Dubbs, Guest, and their authors have provided a much-needed curriculum for the emergency physician. Kudos to the contributors for an outstanding issue that will improve patient care and will certainly ease our stress when managing these patients!

Amal Mattu, MD
Department of Emergency Medicine
University of Maryland School of Medicine
110 South Paca Street
6th Floor, Suite 200
Baltimore, MD 21201, USA

E-mail address:
amattu@som.umaryland.edu

Preface

The Emergency Department Safety Net for Obstetric/Gynecologic Emergencies

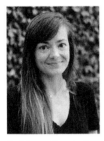 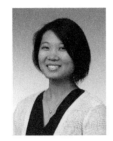

Brittany Guest, DO   Sarah B. Dubbs, MD
Editors

Despite advances in modern medicine, access to obstetric and gynecologic care has declined in many areas across the United States and North America. As a result, we are experiencing a rise in the frequency of obstetric and gynecologic issues requiring attention in the Emergency Department (ED). This important and timely issue of the *Emergency Medicine Clinics of North America* covers cutting-edge literature and updates on gynecologic and obstetric emergencies for which emergency physicians must be prepared to manage.

We chose to focus many of the articles on classic obstetric emergencies, aiming to provide updated information and evidence to guide clinical care. From trauma evaluation, to the assessment and management of surgical emergencies in pregnant patients, cardiovascular and hypertensive emergencies in pregnancy, abortion and miscarriage complications, ED delivery, and an article focused on resuscitation of the obstetric patient, the spectrum of potential complications is covered. In addition, a detailed article on ultrasound in pregnancy discusses the application of point-of-care ultrasound in pregnant or potentially pregnant patients.

In addition to the classic obstetric emergencies, we have also included articles focused on special populations. Articles are focused on adolescent gynecologic emergencies, care of victims of sexual assault and intimate partner violence, care of transgender patients, and considerations in postmenopausal women. The importance of achieving a level of expertise and comfort with these special populations is paramount, particularly in the chaotic environment of the ED.

Included in the issue is a comprehensive article on the care of pregnant patients with COVID virus infection. As the pandemic transitions to an endemic phase and despite the advent of vaccines, pregnant patients remain vulnerable to critical illness from

Emerg Med Clin N Am 41 (2023) xv–xvi
https://doi.org/10.1016/j.emc.2023.02.001
0733-8627/23/© 2023 Published by Elsevier Inc.

infection with SARS-CoV-2. In this scenario, both the mother's and the fetus' morbidity and mortality are at stake, so understanding the pathophysiology and updated management options as they evolve is of even greater importance.

We hope that you find these articles informative and valuable in the clinical care of patients in your practice setting. Whether that setting is a critical access hospital in rural America or a bustling inner-city academic ED, one thing reigns true: our patients rely on us to be their safety net, and we must be ready to care for obstetric and gynecologic emergencies of all ages and types.

We would like to thank the editorial team at Elsevier's *Emergency Medicine Clinics of North America* and our consulting editor, Dr Amal Mattu, for the opportunity to work together on this issue. We would also like to extend our sincere gratitude to each of the authors who contributed to this publication, as it is truly their expertise and hard work that brings this text to life!

Brittany Guest, DO
Department of Emergency Medicine
David Geffen School of Medicine at UCLA
Director of EM:RAPs Live and Virtual Events
Los Angeles, CA 90095, USA

Sarah B. Dubbs, MD
Department of Emergency Medicine
University of Maryland School of Medicine
Baltimore, MD 21201, USA

E-mail addresses:
bjguest44@gmail.com (B. Guest)
sdubbs@som.umaryland.edu (S.B. Dubbs)

Trauma in Pregnancy

Jessica Downing, MD[a], Lucas Sjeklocha, MD[b],*

KEYWORDS

- Pregnancy • Trauma • Resuscitation • Perimortem cesarean delivery
- Physiology of pregnancy

KEY POINTS

- Traumatic injuries during pregnancy are not rare, and they remain the key cause of non-obstetric maternal death.
- Optimal fetal resuscitation depends on optimal maternal resuscitation, and interventions or tests, including computed tomography imaging, should not be withheld during pregnancy if otherwise indicated.
- Perimortem cesarean delivery, also call resuscitative hysterotomy, is indicated within 5 minutes of maternal arrest but may have benefits and potential maternal or fetal survival beyond that time period.
- Physiologic and anatomic changes in pregnancy require modification to resuscitation including relief of aortocaval compression, optimal chest drain placement, and optimal vascular access.
- Cardiotocographic monitoring in only indicated in a potential viable pregnancy.

INTRODUCTION

Trauma in the pregnant patient represents a significant burden of injury and mortality, though it is infrequently encountered in daily practice, approximately one in 12 women experience trauma during pregnancy and it represents the leading cause of nonobstetric maternal death in the United States.[1–3] Despite aggressive public health measures, mortality rates associated with trauma—and especially with motor vehicle collisions—are increasing worldwide.[4] In the United States, most of the injuries sustained during pregnancy are due to blunt trauma, with a minority caused by penetrating mechanisms and burns. Pregnancy remains a vulnerable state, both because of socioeconomic factors and physiologic factors that alter the spectrum of injury.[5]

[a] R Adams Cowley Shock Trauma Center, University of Maryland Medical Center, 22 South Greene Street, Baltimore, MD 21201, USA; [b] Department of Emergency Medicine, Program in Trauma, R Adams Cowley Shock Trauma Center, University of Maryland, School of Medicine, 22 South Greene Street, Baltimore, MD 21201, USA
* Corresponding author.
E-mail address: lsjeklocha@som.umaryland.edu

Emerg Med Clin N Am 41 (2023) 223–245
https://doi.org/10.1016/j.emc.2022.12.001
0733-8627/23/© 2022 Elsevier Inc. All rights reserved.

emed.theclinics.com

The pregnant patient presenting to the emergency department with an acute trauma constitutes a worrisome population for the emergency physician, given the presence of two patients, and the risk of both fetal and maternal injury. Studies have poor correlation between prehospital mechanism and maternal and fetal injury, and all injuries should be approached with vigilance.[2] A team-based approach with clear leadership has been shown in some studies to improve processes of care and patient outcomes.[6,7] The team may include representatives from emergency medicine, trauma surgery, obstetrics and gynecology, anesthesia, neonatology, pediatrics, and pediatric surgery. The emergency physician should serve as team leader and take responsibility for prioritizing and coordinating multiple teams and interests in care. The increased cognitive load associated with these scenarios provides additional challenges.

In all trauma patients, the initial assessment begins with a structured and swift evaluation focusing on addressing life-threatening compromise airway, breathing, and circulation.[8] The resuscitation of pregnant trauma patients follows similar principles, with some additions and deviations. The initial focus should be on maternal resuscitation; the fetus depends on maternal well-being, so the best treatment for the fetus is initial maternal resuscitation and stabilization.[9–11] Clear maternal indications for imaging should generally take precedence over concern about potential fetal harm.[5,12,13] Pregnancy may not always be evident to the team or the patient, and universal screening with urine or blood should be implemented.[14]

EPIDEMIOLOGY

Trauma is the leading cause of nonobstetric maternal death.[2,3] In a patient-level review of one US states' traumatic injuries, 4.6% of trauma admissions were pregnant, and approximately 0.4% of fetal deaths were attributed to trauma.[15] A study of trauma patients at a level 1 trauma center found incidental pregnancy in 0.3% of total admissions and 11.0% of all pregnant patients.[14] Most pregnant trauma patients are injured through blunt mechanisms; motor vehicle injuries represent the most prevalent mechanism, followed by falls, assaults (including gunshot wounds), and burns.[5] Pregnant patients, particularly in the third trimester, are at over a 1.6 times higher risk of injury than similarly matched nonpregnant patients.[15] The prevalence of intimate partner violence is estimated to be greater than 8% during pregnancy[8,16]; estimates are made difficult by significant underreporting, underrecognition, and decreased likelihood of seeking medical care.[17,18]

Injuries during pregnancy can results in significant adverse maternal and fetal outcomes, including up to a 37.7% risk of delivery during the index hospitalization.[2,5,19,20] Although major trauma lead to the highest incidence of adverse fetal and maternal outcomes, so-called minor traumas account for a large number of adverse pregnancy outcomes as well.[21]

ZERO POINT SURVEY: MOBILIZING RESOURCES

When possible, all pregnant trauma patients should be evaluated at a designated trauma center with in-house labor and delivery and neonatology teams. If the team receives advanced notice that a pregnant patient is en route for the evaluation of trauma, the on-call obstetrician should be called to the trauma bay and the neonatal intensive care unit should be placed on alert. The trauma and obstetric team should discuss any information provided by emergency medical services and discuss key action items of their plan. Bedside tools and checklists can assist with management. In addition to standard trauma equipment and an ultrasound machine, fetal monitoring equipment and materials required for an emergency C-section should be brought to the trauma bay. Fetal monitoring belts may be laid out on the stretcher in advance to facilitate prompt initiation of cardiotocographic monitoring with minimal disruption to the trauma survey.[22]

PRIMARY SURVEY
Airway

Physiologic changes of pregnancy
Pregnant patients often have increased mucosal edema, rhinitis, and congestion with hyperemia that predisposes to bleeding as well as increased Mallampati score.[23,24] These changes make airway management more difficult and increase likelihood of failed intubations.[25–28] The relative increase in aspiration risk and need for increased oxygen delivery makes earlier definitive airway more desirable in pregnancy. Decreased functional residual capacity (FRC), impaired venous return in the supine position, and fetal intolerance of hypoxia contribute to the physiologic difficulties in airway management (**Table 1**).[25,26,29]

Intubation
Airway management in pregnancy is associated with the increased difficulty of laryngoscopy, decreased oxygen reserve, and heightened risk of aspiration.[25,28,30] A review of obstetric anesthesia found approximately one in 390 attempts at intubation result in a failed airway.[25]

Rapid sequence induction and intubation is pregnancy follows similar principles of high-risk airway management with a special emphasis on positioning, preoxygenation, and airway edema (**Box 1**). Physicians should consider preoxygenation with head of bed elevation during laryngoscopy and optimize functional residual capacity and

Table 1	
Relevant physiologic changes in pregnancy	
Head, Ears, Eyes, Nose and Throat (HEENT)	Increased mucosal edema Increased mucosal friability Relative swelling of the tongue
Respiratory	Elevation of the diaphragm Respiratory alkalosis Decreased expiratory reserve volume
Cardiovascular	Increased cardiac output Increased oxygen delivery Increased blood volume Decreased blood pressure in 2nd trimester Aortocaval compression beginning at 20 wk
Gastrointestinal	Decreased lower esophageal sphincter tone Delayed gastric emptying Intestinal shift from gravid uterus
Genitourinary	Physiologic hydronephrosis Decreased serum bicarbonate
Hematologic	Increased red blood cell mass Physiologic anemia due to increased total blood volume Hypercoagulable state Increase in clotting factors, including fibrinogen
Musculoskeletal	Ligamentous laxity Change in center of gravity Increased fall risk

> **Box 1**
> **Airway management considerations**
>
> Goal oxygen saturation >95%
>
> Standard rapid sequence intubation (RSI) medications can be used in pregnancy
>
> Anticipate increased airway difficulty
>
> Consider video laryngoscopy due to potential visualization difficulty and neck stabilization
>
> Smaller endotracheal tubes may be required (6.0, 6.5, 7.0)
>
> Meticulous preoxygenation
>
> Elevation of the head of bed 30°
>
> Consider cricoid pressure and preinduction NGT due to aspiration risk
>
> Prepare for a surgical airway

maintain longer safe apnea times before intubation.[30,31] Gastric decompression with placement of a nasogastric tube before intubation has been recommended due to decreased gastroinestinal (GI) transit time and gastric emptying combined with decreased lower esophageal sphincter tone increase the risk of vomiting and aspiration.[23,32–34] Cricoid pressure may also be considered to prevent passive aspiration; however, it is difficult to delivery optimal pressure without airway compression.[25] Avoid unnecessary airway manipulation and blind intubation due to bleeding risk.

Standard RSI medications can be used safely during pregnancy. When selecting equipment, physicians should consider video laryngoscopy if it is available and have smaller endotracheal tubes (down to a 6.0) and a bougie readily available. Consider the potential increased risk of a surgical airway and have resources available.

Breathing

Physiologic changes of pregnancy

During pregnancy, the maternal respiratory and cardiovascular systems undergo changes designed to oxygen delivery to the fetus. Progesterone and estrogen, among other hormones, lead to increased respiratory rate and tidal volumes, which reduce $PaCO_2$ to 25 to 32 mm Hg and increase PaO_2 to 104 to 108 mm Hg, leading to a respiratory alkalosis with a typical arterial pH of 7.40 to 7.45 and increased oxygen delivery.[12,23,32] The gravid uterus elevates the diaphragm 3 to 5 cm with anteroposterior and transverse expansion of the chest wall but overall reductions in total lung capacity and functional residual capacity.[30,35,36] Because of these changes, maternal decompensation may be imminent or ongoing despite normal pH, PaO_2, and $PaCO_2$, and desaturation may occur quickly and be difficult to reverse.[5,25] The rib cage also remodels and becomes more compliant, potentially decreasing the risk of risk fracture without changing the risk of intrathoracic injury[36,37]; significant pulmonary injury may occur without rib fractures.[37]

Mechanical ventilation

If mechanical ventilation is instituted, an oxygen saturation of greater than 95% should be targeted to support fetal oxygenation.[9,10] The goal PCO_2 should be approximately 32 mm Hg.[38] It is important to avoid both underventilation and overventilation as PCO_2 less than 30 mm Hg has been associated with decreased uterine blood flow, whereas hypercapnia is associated with fetal acidosis.

Chest tubes
The diaphragm will be displaced superiorly as pregnancy advances, changing anatomic landmarks for chest tubes or needle decompression and complicating physical examination.[12] Chest tubes should be placed one or two spaces higher than in the nonpregnant patient, typically above the fourth intercostal space.[39]

Circulation

Physiologic changes of pregnancy
Pregnancy is a state of relative hypervolemia to facilitate fetal oxygen delivery; vital signs and characteristics of venous return evolve throughout the course of pregnancy. By approximately 8 weeks gestation, plasma volume begins to expand up to 45% with a concomitant increase in cardiac output.[12,40] Cardiac output will increase 30% to 50% by the third trimester.[32] Heart rate increases an expected 15 to 20 beats per minute. Blood pressure change is characterized by an initial decrease in diastolic blood pressure by (10–15 mm Hg) during the second trimester and subsequent increase toward normal in the third trimester.[23,32] This increased cardiac output helps to supply the expanding uterus and support the fetus.

As the uterus expands, it exerts a mass effect on the local vasculature. Inferior vena cava (IVC) compression in late pregnancy reduces venous return and cardiac output by up to 30%.[12,23,33,41,42] Alterations to blood vessels during pregnancy may increase both the risk of clotting due to a hypercoagulable state and a greater risk of dissection or injury due to hormonal changes.[1]

Inferior vena cava offloading techniques and vascular access
Strategies to mitigate compression of the IVC in gravid trauma patients are critical to improve circulation.[1,8,10,12] These include manual left lateral uterine displacement or elevation of the right hip to improve venous return. Because of the compression of the IVC by the gravid uterus, the upper extremities are preferred for large bore peripheral or central venous access.

Transfusion and massive transfusion protocol (MTP)
The hypervolemia of pregnancy creates a relative tolerance to the expected hemorrhage of childbirth but may mask hemorrhage in traumatic injuries; maternal blood loss can reach 1500 mL before significant signs appear. Initial resuscitation may include up to 1 L of warmed crystalloid.[33] Immediate blood transfusion is appropriate in patient with suspected or overt hemorrhage with activation of massive transfusion for those in shock.[9,12,43,44] Type O-negative blood should be requested if type-specific is not available to avoid alloimmunization.[9] Optimal transfusion ratios of packed red blood cells, fresh-frozen plasma, and platelets are likely unchanged in pregnancy; a 1:1:1 approach is recommended. Vasopressors reduce uterine blood flow and should be avoided until hypovolemia and ongoing blood loss has been corrected.[45]

Resuscitative endovascular balloon occlusion of the aorta
Resuscitative endovascular balloon occlusion of the aorta (REBOA) has been successfully used to temporize bleeding due to severe non-traumatic obstetric hemorrhage en route to surgical intervention. There has been one published case report detailing the utilization of REBOA in the management of severe hemorrhagic shock in the setting of uterine rupture and fetal demise secondary to an abdominal gunshot wound.[46] Of note, fetal death had been confirmed before the patient's resuscitation. The balloon was initially inflated in zone 1; it was moved to zone 3 intraoperatively, after delivery of the fetus and before uterine artery ligation. The patient survived to hospital discharge.

Traumatic Cardiac Arrest

Traumatic cardiac arrest in pregnancy should prompt rapid identification and intervention on reversible causes (such as hemorrhage, tension pneumothorax, cardiac tamponade, and hypoxia), recognition of pregnancy and estimation of gestational age, assessment of signs of life, adjunctive maneuvers to restore maternal circulation, and evaluation for perimortem cesarean delivery (PMCD).[47,48] The gravid uterus should be immediately manually displaced to the left, and all patients should receive supplemental oxygen, a secured definitive airway, large bore intravenous (IV) access above the diaphragm, balanced blood resuscitation, and empiric bilateral finger thoracostomies.[8,12,49] Although there is little evidence in this population, at this time accepted indications for resuscitative thoracotomy in the nonpregnant patient should be applied in pregnancy, with assessment of signs of life, mechanism, and timing of arrest as well as local resources guiding the decision.[39,50,51] Available resources including trauma surgery, obstetrics, anesthesia, and pediatrics or neonatology along with appropriate resuscitative equipment should be mobilized, ideally with a bundled activation system.[42]

The approach to cardiopulmonary resuscitation (CPR), defibrillation, epinephrine, and other drug administration during medical cardiac arrest is unchanged during pregnancy.[8,42,52,53] Although it is not always possible to differentiate traumatic from non-traumatic causes, the evidence for CPR and epinephrine in traumatic arrest remain conflicting and unclear.[49,54,55]

Perimortem cesarean delivery

PMCD, also termed resuscitative hysterotomy, may confer benefit on both mother and fetus in the setting of maternal extremis.[29,42,49,56] If standard resuscitation fails, PMCD may relieve aortocaval compression from the gravid uterus and allow fetal resuscitation. PMCD should be performed within 5 minutes if initial maternal resuscitation is unsuccessful and either the fetus is deemed potentially viable or the uterus is above the umbilicus, which is associated with aortocaval compression.[39,42,49,51,53] The assessment of fetal viability (typically defined as 23–24 weeks gestation or greater) may be obtained based on history, examination (suggested by a with the gravid uterus palpable 2 cm above the umbilicus), or by bedside ultrasound evaluation.[10,39,49,57] The procedure is not intended to be sterile, requires limited equipment, and can be performed in austere environments; the goal is to remove the fetus, begin fetal resuscitation, and evacuate and displace of the uterus for maternal benefit.[56,58,59]

Prompt PMCD has been associated with improved maternal and fetal outcomes; PMCD within 5 minutes was associated fetal survival with 95% survival in one study.[60,61] Cases of infant survival with improvement in material hemodynamics and maternal return of spontaneous circulation have been described beyond 15 minutes of arrest; one survey of published reports described an average time to delivery of 14 minutes.[59–64]

SECONDARY SURVEY
Focused History: AMPLE and CODE

The acronym AMPLE is a well-known roadmap used to guide focused history taking for trauma patients: allergies, medications, past medical and surgical history, last oral intake, and events leading up to injury (**Fig. 1**). In the pregnant patient, a focused obstetric history should be taken as well. One set of authors have suggested the acronym CODE, reminding clinicians to inquire into (1) complications of pregnancy,

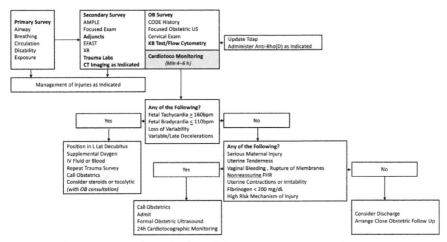

Fig. 1. Initial assessment and monitoring of the pregnant trauma patient.

(2) obstetric history and primary prenatal care provider, (3) dates, including dating method, and (4) obstetric symptoms during and since the event, including vaginal bleeding, contractions, leakage of fluid, and fetal movements.[22] Special care should be taken to identify obstetric complications that may interfere with or complicate assessment and resuscitation after trauma (such as preeclampsia, which is associated with already reduced intravascular volume) or emergency C-section (such as prior surgeries that may have resulted in scarring).[9]

The Physical Examination

The physical examination of the pregnant trauma patient should not differ significantly from that of the non-trauma patient and should follow Advanced Trauma Life Support guidelines.[9] The interpretation of physical examination findings, however, may vary slightly. Assessing for signs of peritonitis is an integral part of the trauma physical examination; however, during pregnancy the peritoneum stretches and becomes relatively desensitized. This, combined with the gravid uterus's position anterior in the abdomen, makes patients less likely to exhibit rebound or guarding even in the setting of peritoneal violation.[1,45] Moreover, the pressure of the uterus on the more posterior vasculature and organs leads to a relative venous hypertension, which increases the risk of bleeding.[65]

The uterus itself is likely to bear a significant amount of the force transmitted in abdominal injuries. Whereas abdominal tenderness often raises concern for bowel perforation in trauma patients, tenderness over the uterus should raise concern for placental abruption.[9] Owing to the upward displacement of abdominal organs by the growing uterus, the abdominal cavity extends farther cranially in pregnant than nonpregnant women; the abdominal cavity should be considered to start at fourth intercostal space and the tip of the scapula.[9] This essentially expands the thoracoabdominal area where penetrating trauma can injure both thoracic and abdominal organs.

An internal vaginal examination should be included in the secondary survey for all pregnant patients to evaluate for vaginal bleeding, pooling of fluid, and cervical dilation.[9] After 23 weeks gestation, an ultrasound must be performed before speculum or bimanual examination to exclude the presence of placenta previa.

Obstetric Evaluation and Monitoring

Cardiotocographic monitoring

Cardiotocographic monitoring is the most sensitive tool for the diagnosis of placental abruption, which is the leading cause of fetal demise following trauma. Trauma and obstetric guidelines recommend that all pregnant women who suffer trauma after 20-week gestation undergo cardiotocographic monitoring for at least 6 hours.[9,10] A non-reassuring fetal heart rate pattern (including bradycardia $\leq$ 110 bpm, tachycardia $\geq$ 160 bpm, and variable decelerations) should prompt clinicians to reposition the patient in left lateral decubitus, administer additional supplemental oxygen, and resuscitate with additional IV fluids or blood.[9,13] Admission with obstetric consultation, formal obstetric ultrasound, and cardiotocographic monitoring for at least 24 hours should be recommended if any of the following are identified: serious maternal injury, uterine tenderness, vaginal bleeding or rupture of membranes (ROMs), a non-reassuring fetal heart rate pattern, uterine contractions or irritability, fibrinogen less than 200 mg/dL, or a high-risk mechanism of injury.[9,10,66]

Placental abruption has been (rarely) reported over 24 hours after trauma, though the current literature suggests this diagnosis has been foreshadowed by at least one contraction over any 10 minute period during initial monitoring.[17] A small case series of 71 pregnant trauma patients found that no patients with a negative Kleihauer–Betke (KB) test experienced contractions during 4 hours of tocographic monitoring or went on to have preterm labor during their hospitalization, leading the authors to suggest that the duration of cardiotocographic monitoring may be safely limited in the setting of negative KB test.[67]

DIAGNOSTICS
Laboratories

Interpretation in the setting of pregnancy

Complete blood count. During pregnancy, patients experience a "physiologic anemia," reaching an expected decrease in hematocrit to 31% to 35% during late pregnancy. Red blood cell mass increases 20% to 30% in pregnancy and plasma volume 45%, which increases blood volume and adapts for peripartum blood loss.[12,23,32] Hormonal changes are also associated with a leukocytosis up to 14,000 in normal pregnancy and 30,000 during delivery.[23]

Coagulation panel. Maternal coagulation becomes biased toward a relatively procoagulant state with increases in nearly all clotting factors including fibrinogen (with a mean in pregnancy of 450 mg/dL), increased d-dimer, and overall increased thromboembolic risk.[12,68] Low fibrinogen (<200 mg/dL) has been identified as an independent risk factor for critical obstetric hemorrhage[69] and should be considered an indication for admission.[9]

Basic metabolic panel. Increased cardiac output during pregnancy is accompanied by an increase with renal blood flow and glomerular filtration rate.[23,32] This results in an expected decrease in serum creatinine and blood urea nitrogen. The respiratory alkalosis of pregnancy is compensated with a decreased serum bicarbonate level to approximately 19 to 20.

Type and screen. A type and screen should be obtained for all pregnant patients presenting after trauma, even if it is considered minor. Identification of the patients' Rh type will guide the administration of Rh immunoglobulin as prophylaxis against alloimmunization.

Kleihauer–Betke test and flow cytometry

EAST guidelines recommend that KB test be included in the trauma evaluation for all pregnant women greater than 12-week gestation.[10] The KB test screens maternal blood for fetal hemoglobin that has crossed the placenta and entered into maternal systemic circulation, indicating fetomaternal hemorrhage. The traditional use of the test has been to guide the administration of Rh-immunoglobulin to Rh-negative mothers for the prevention of fetal hydrops from Rh-sensitization in future pregnancies.[39] Maternal hemoglobinopathies that raise the percentage of fetal hemoglobin (HbF) in maternal blood in the absence of fetomaternal hemorrhage, such as sickle cell anemia, may result in a false-positive KB test.[70] Flow cytometry and fluorescence microscopy have been suggested as more accurate alternatives to the KB test, though availability may vary.[67,70,71]

Recent literature has suggested that a positive KB test or flow cytometry may, on their own, be a useful indicator of injury severity and predictor of adverse pregnancy outcomes including preterm labor.[72,73] A single-center retrospective study of 71 pregnant women requiring evaluation at a trauma center found that over half of those with a positive KB test — and none of those with a negative KB test — went on to have preterm labor.[67] For this reason, it is recommended for all pregnancies, rather than only those of Rh-negative mothers.

Imaging

Point-of-care ultrasound

The focused assessment with sonography in trauma (FAST) examination has become an essential tool used to evaluate the unstable patient presenting after blunt trauma. The sensitivity of FAST has been reported to be lower in pregnant patients (approximately 60%) than in nonpregnant patients and is best in the first trimester.[17,74] Specificity is still very good (94%).[17,74] Although the presence of a small amount of pelvic free fluid is often considered physiologic in pregnancy (and in women of reproductive age in general), all free fluid should be presumed pathologic in the setting of trauma and should prompt additional assessment with computed tomography (CT) imaging or operative exploration, depending on the clinical scenario.[74] As with all patients, a negative FAST does not "rule out" intraperitoneal hemorrhage but should rather prompt investigation for other sources of hypotension in an unstable patient or further evaluation with serial examinations or CT in a stable patient. Per American College of Obstetrics and Gynecology (ACOG)' recommendations, ultrasound has not been associated with risk to the pregnant patient or fetus, though use of this imaging modality should still comply with the principles of "ALARA": the use of a "dose" "as low as reasonably achievable" to answer the relevant clinical question at hand.[13]

The bedside performance of the FAST examination presents an opportunity for an initial evaluation of the pregnancy. Using ultrasound, clinicians can quickly confirm the number of fetuses, evaluate for intrauterine fetal demise, and estimate gestational age by measuring the gestational sac, crown-rump length, femur length, or biparietal diameter, depending on the stage of pregnancy. This will help guide additional obstetric evaluation and monitoring and inform additional procedures that may be required. Clinicians should also identify the location of the placenta to evaluate for placenta previa. Although all pregnant trauma patients should be evaluated for vaginal bleeding, a bimanual or speculum examination should be deferred until placenta previa has been ruled out. The diagnosis of placenta previa is also essential in anticipation of possible preterm labor induced by trauma. Finally, the FAST examination provides an opportunity for a quick initial assessment of fetal heart rate and subjective assessment of amniotic fluid volume (small, normal, or large). This quick glimpse into fetal well-being will inform the urgency with which additional obstetric evaluation or intervention is required. Sonography should not be relied on to evaluate for placental abruption, as the sensitivity has been reported to be unacceptably low.[75] Large clots visualized in the uterus should raise significant concern for abruption.[75]

X-ray and computed tomography: considerations regarding radiation exposure. X-ray and CT imaging are mainstays of the trauma evaluation. Both require the use of ionizing radiation. The impact of ionizing radiation on pregnancy and fetal development depends on the "dose" of fetal radiation and the stage of fetal development at which it is encountered. Fetal radiation "dose" is determined by both the amount of radiation generated during any single test and the anatomic location at which it is directed in the pregnant patient–for example, a maternal pelvic CT will result in a higher fetal radiation dose than a chest CT (**Table 2**[10,13,76]).[13] During the first 2 weeks of pregnancy, ionizing radiation of greater than 5 to 10 rad (50–100 mGy) may result in pregnancy loss.[13,77] During weeks 2 to 8, doses greater than 20 rad may result in growth restriction or congenital anomalies.[13,77] After 8 weeks, the primary risk is of intellectual disability; early in pregnancy (before 16 weeks), the risk of intellectual disability is higher and occurs at lower doses of fetal radiation (>6 rad as opposed to >25 rad).[13,77] Exposure to less than 5 rad has not been associated with pregnancy loss or increased teratogenesis.[10] The risk of cancer associated with in-utero radiation exposure is thought to be low.[13] The lifetime risk of cancer development in a neonate is expected to be increased by 0.4% per 1 rad of exposure.[77] It is not known how this translates to in-utero exposure.

Most of the diagnostic imaging procedures, individually, do not approach a fetal radiation dose associated with pregnancy loss or adverse effects on fetal development.[13] Professional guidelines (Eastern Association for the Surgery of Trauma (EAST), ACOG, and Society of Obstetricians and Gynaegologists of Canada (SOGC)) emphasize that diagnostic studies, including imaging, should not be delayed or deferred when clinically indicated due to concerns regarding fetal exposure to radiation.[10,13,39] Shielding of the uterus during select scans is not recommended.[78,79] Furthermore, iodinated intravenous contrast should not be withheld if clinically indicated for diagnostic purposes.[13] There are few circumstances in trauma—such as

Table 2
Expected fetal radiation dose associated with imaging techniques typically used in the evaluation of moderate to severe trauma[10,13,76]

Imaging Study	Fetal Radiation Exposure (Rads)
X-Rays	
Chest X-ray	0.000025–0.0005
Pelvis X-ray	0.04
Abdominal X-ray	0.01–0.03
Extremity X-ray	<0.0011
CT Scans	
CT head	0.0011–0.01
CT neck	<0.0001–0.01
CT chest	0.001–0.066
CT abdomen	0.13–3.5
CT pelvis	1–5
Sum: Trauma "Pan Scan"	1.13–8.59

that of spinal cord injury (SCI)—in which MRI is the diagnostic modality of choice. MRI has not been associated with adverse effects during pregnancy, though should not be relied on as an alternative outside of these circumstances due to the risk of significant delay in diagnosis of life-threatening injuries. The use of gadolinium contrast in pregnancy is controversial but is also not typically indicated in evaluation for trauma.[13]

CARE AFTER INITIAL RESUSCITATION
Prophylaxis

All pregnant patients presenting with trauma should receive tetanus prophylaxis if vaccination is not up to date.[80] Routine administration of Anti-D Rh immunoglobulin is recommended for all Rh-negative pregnant patients presenting with trauma, even in the face of a negative KB or flow cytometry test.[9] A single dose of 300 mg is sufficient in most (90%) cases and will neutralize 30 mL of fetal blood if given within 72 hours.[9,67,70] Larger fetomaternal hemorrhage requires proportionately higher doses.

Cefazolin, commonly used for prophylaxis in patients with contaminated open wounds or fractures, is considered safe in pregnancy (Category B).[81] Aminoglycosides, including gentamicin, carry a black-box warning for congenital deafness after in-utero exposure and should be avoided in pregnant patients. Ceftriaxone and metronidazole, often used empirically in the setting of bowel perforation, are both considered safe in pregnancy (Category B).

Blunt Trauma

Operative management of injuries
The decision to proceed with operative management of abdominal injuries should not be significantly impacted by the presence of pregnancy.[71] There is little evidence to date regarding the use of endovascular therapies in the treatment of trauma among pregnant patients. Case reports have described successful splenic artery embolization for grade III to V splenic injury in the setting of pregnancy and blunt trauma, which is thought to minimize the risk of preterm delivery associated with open surgery.[74,82–84] Endovascular specialists, such as vascular surgery or interventional radiology, may be mobilized for pregnant trauma patients as for nonpregnant patients with similar injuries.

Delivery
Operative management of injuries does not necessitate delivery. Nonetheless, it is recommended that an obstetrician be present in the operating room to assist with delivery if needed as well as repair of any injuries to the reproductive organs. Delivery should be considered in the case of maternal hemorrhagic shock or arrest, fetal demise, or if the gravid uterus prevents necessary repair of other injuries.[71] Unstable thoracolumbar spinal injuries have been suggested as an indication for delivery as well.[71] Pelvic fractures should not prelude continuation of pregnancy to term or vaginal delivery.[71] If delivery is anticipated, neonatology should be contacted as soon as possible.

Penetrating Trauma

Operative management of injuries
All patients with penetrating trauma should be immediately evaluated by a trauma surgeon and obstetrician immediately. There is very little evidence available regarding the management of penetrating trauma in pregnancy and almost none in the past 40 years. Much of the existing literature focuses on penetrating trauma to the abdomen. Although maternal mortality is reported to be very low,[45] fetal mortality is high and

impacted primarily by gestational age at the time of injury.[84] It is thought that the gravid uterus essentially acts as a "shield"; once it occupies space as an intra-abdominal organ, the uterus is more likely than other organs to be impacted by penetrating injury, particularly if the injury site is anterior, and is thought to absorb much of the force associated with missile wounds.[45] Visceral injury in the setting of stab wounds has been reported to be 50% less common in pregnant women than their nonpregnant counterparts.[39] Upper abdominal wounds carry a higher risk of peritoneal violation.[39] Intuitively, gunshot wounds are associated with poorer maternal and fetal outcomes than stab wounds.[85]

In the case of penetrating trauma, the indications for immediate operative intervention are unchanged from those applied to nonpregnant patients. In some cases, it has been suggested that stable patients may be managed nonoperatively if they have a benign abdominal examination, negative digital rectal examination, no hematuria, and an identified wound below the uterine fundus, and the missile is visualized in the uterine cavity on imaging, though again, available evidence is limited.[86]

Delivery

Infant survival has not been associated with maternal injury severity or distress in the case of penetrating injury. C-section is likely warranted if the gestational age is ≥ 26 weeks and fetal heart tones are appreciated.[87] If the mother is not in extremis, emergency C-section is not typically recommended in a preterm pregnancy, unless an injury to the fetus, cord, or placenta is thought to be the source of maternal hemorrhage or precludes the fetus from receiving appropriate blood and oxygen, or the gravid uterus interferes with the surgeons ability to manage other injuries in need of repair.[45] In the case of IUFD, induction and delivery after the acute management of trauma is recommended.[45] Case reports have described successful delivery maternal gunshot wound to the abdomen during the third trimester, with operative intervention for the neonate required following delivery.[84,88] These patients were ultimately discharged from the hospital with good outcomes at follow-up. Based on available evidence, however, such outcomes are rare.

Obstetric Complications

Placental abruption

Placental abruption is the most common obstetric injury following trauma and can occur in the setting of otherwise minor injuries.[9] Force that is absorbed by the relatively elastic and muscular uterus is then passed on to the placenta, which is much more rigid—this transmission creates a shearing force between the two that leads to abruption.[71] Placental abruption should be considered for any pregnant patient with abdominal pain, uterine tenderness, contractions, or vaginal bleeding after trauma.[9,71] It may be an inciting factor for disseminated intravascular coagulation and should be suspected in any pregnant trauma patient with low fibrinogen (<200 mg/dL).[71] It is best diagnosed with cardiotocographic monitoring, though some studies have described good sensitivity and specificity with CT scan in specialized centers.[89] Ultrasound has poor sensitivity and specificity and should not be relied on to make this diagnosis. Abruption usually occurs within hours of the trauma, leading to the recommendation for cardiotocographic monitoring for 4 to 6 hours after hospital arrival. Although delayed abruption has been reported, it is almost always heralded by uterine contractions on tocographic monitoring.

Placental abruption is, in most circumstances, an indication for emergent delivery in a viable pregnancy; abruption is associated with high fetal mortality, which can be reduced significantly by prompt C-section if the fetus is viable at the time of injury.[9,39]

Once diagnosed in an otherwise stable patient, placental abruption should prompt immediate preparation for transfer to the obstetric operating room for emergency delivery via C-section.[9] Although a vaginal delivery may be acceptable in select cases, emergency providers should presume that placental abruption in a viable pregnancy is an indication for emergent C-section unless informed otherwise by the consulting obstetrician.

Uterine rupture
Uterine rupture is rare but deadly, associated with high maternal mortality rates and fetal mortality approaching 100%.[9] Prior C-section is an important risk factor.[71] It should be considered in unstable patients as well as those with peritonitis, abnormal uterine contour or palpable fetal parts, noted ascent of the fetal presenting part, or a sudden negative change in fetal heart tracing.[9] Once diagnosed, uterine rupture is an indication for immediate laparotomy, delivery, and uterine repair or hysterectomy.[9,71]

Premature rupture of membranes and preterm labor
Trauma is an important risk factor for premature ROMs and preterm labor.[71] Patients who are unable to participate in history and examination should be evaluated for leakage of amniotic fluid with a sterile speculum examination after first excluding placenta previa with ultrasound. The treatment for premature ROM and preterm labor in trauma is not significantly different from that in the non-trauma patient.[71]

SPECIAL CIRCUMSTANCES
Burns

Burns in pregnancy are relatively rare in high-income countries. Data regarding the management of burns in pregnancy are limited, arising primarily from small case series and case reports. Evidence comparing outcomes of pregnant and nonpregnant burn victims is conflicting.[90] The total body surface area (TBSA) affected by burn and the presence of inhalation injury have been identified as the most significant indicator of poor outcomes for mother and fetus; minor burns have relatively little impact on mother or pregnancy, but larger burns carry significant morbidity and mortality. Prior studies have estimated that burns greater than 25% TBSA are associated with a 48% mortality,[90] and those greater than 40% to 50% carry a mortality rate approaching 100%.[17,91]

Airway
Later trimesters of pregnancy are associated with an increase in airway edema and decreased pulmonary reserve, making patients particularly susceptible to respiratory failure and airway compromise in the setting of inhalation injury or facial burns.[92] Clinicians should have a low threshold to intubate these patients and should anticipate a difficult airway.

Breathing
Owing to the risk of fetal hypoxia from poor placental perfusion in the setting of increased capillary permeability and distributive shock from burns, it is recommended that all pregnant burn victims be treated with supplemental oxygen, even in the absence of inhalation injury.[93] Those requiring intubation and mechanical ventilation due to presumed inhalation injury should be evaluated with bronchoscopy shortly after intubation.[93]

Circulation
Prompt and aggressive fluid resuscitation is recommended for pregnant burn patients. Owing to increased circulating blood volume and decreased systemic vascular

resistance, as well as an increase in TBSA, may mask hypovolemia and increase the risk of under-resuscitation when using the Parkland formula and other standard guidelines for fluid resuscitation. It is recommended that fluid resuscitation be tailored to individual needs based on urine output, vital signs, and fetal heart rate.[92]

Disability

All burn victims should be evaluated for carbon monoxide (CO) toxicity. CO toxicity is associated with significant maternal and fetal mortality as well as fetal anatomic malformations or neurologic derangements as the result of hypoxia.[94] All patients with suspected or confirmed CO toxicity should be treated with 100% oxygen via non-rebreather. Based on the limited animal studies, it is recommended that oxygen therapy be continued five times longer than needed to resolve maternal COHb.[95] Any patient with neurologic symptoms, signs of fetal hypoxia or distress, or COHb greater than 20% should receive hyperbaric oxygen therapy.[94,96]

Exposure

Most pregnant patients can be treated with usual burn care, including tetanus prophylaxis, topical antimicrobials, and moist occlusive dressings.[93] Systemic antibiotics should not be administered prophylactically. Debridement, escharotomy, surgical excision, and skin grafting should be performed if indicated as soon as the patient's clinical condition allows. Data from case series suggest that early surgical wound excision may reduce time to normalization of hemodynamics and improve fetal and maternal outcomes.[97]

Pain control

Multimodal pain control is an essential component of burn management. Oral or intravenous acetaminophen is a mainstay of treatment. Although non-steroidal anti-inflammatory drug (NSAID) are commonly used for pain management in burn patients, they are associated with miscarriage early in pregnancy as well as early patent ductus arteriosus (PDA) closure in the third trimester[98] and oligohydramnios after 20 weeks[99] and should thus be avoided in pregnant patients. Opioids, including patient-controlled analgesia, have been shown to be safe in burn care and are recommended for pregnant burn patients.[92,100] Case reports have also suggested that ketamine (started at 10 mg/h and titrated to a maximum dose of 1 mg/kg/h)[101] and epidural administration of regional anesthesia and narcotics[102] may be effectively used as an adjunct for pain management in pregnant patients with burns.

Obstetric care

Obstetric care in the setting of burns highly depends on the stage of pregnancy and TBSA affected by burns. Continuous fetal monitoring and tocodynamometry should be initiated for all patients with viable pregnancies; sterile covers should be used if the monitors may overly burned skin.[92] Before 34 weeks gestation and certainly before 28 weeks, steroids and tocolytics should be administered to delay delivery if the mother's physiologic state allows for safe continuation of pregnancy (**Fig. 2**).[90,92,93] Magnesium may be the preferred tocolytic agent in the setting of burns due to relatively fewer hemodynamic and metabolic effects.[93] In the setting of maternal instability or significant burns later in pregnancy, delivery via induction of labor or emergency C-section is indicated. Intubation and mechanical ventilation is not a contraindication to labor and vaginal delivery, if the mother's hemodynamics permits.[93]

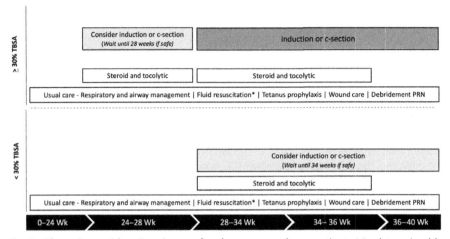

Fig. 2. Obstetric considerations in care for the pregnant burn patient. *As determined by individualized goals.

Traumatic Brain Injury

Evidence regarding traumatic brain injury (TBI) in pregnant patients is extremely sparse. There are no established guidelines or recommendations for care of the pregnant patients with TBI.[103] Many epidemiological data on blunt head injuries in pregnancy are over 20 year old; in 1992, it was estimated that 9.1% of maternal deaths due to trauma in pregnancy were the result of blunt head injury.[3] The spectrum of effects of TBI on the mother and fetus are largely unknown. A retrospective study of the National Trauma Data Bank found a trend toward increased mortality among pregnant patients compared with nonpregnant female TBI patients, though their findings did not reach statistical significance.[104] This study suggests that prior hypotheses that increased progesterone levels in pregnancy might be neuroprotective in the setting of TBI are likely incorrect.

Airway

In the setting of altered mental status, it may be necessary to secure the airway early to avoid hypopnea and aspiration, for which pregnant patients are already at increased risk due to reduced lower esophageal tone.[105] Again, this should be anticipated to be a potentially difficult intubation.

Breathing

Hypoxia is associated with worsening of neurologic injury as well as poor fetal outcomes. Hypercapnia and hypocapnia carry risk to mother and fetus in the setting of TBI and should be avoided: normocapnia should be targeted if at all possible.

Circulation

Continuous fetal heart monitoring should be implemented as soon as possible and maintained throughout the acute phase of injury. Clinicians should take active measures to avoid hypotension, a secondary insult associated with worsening of injury, and to which pregnant women (and their fetuses) are particularly vulnerable.[103] Hypertension may be deleterious as well due to increases in intracranial pressure (ICP). If vasopressors are required, phenylephrine is recommended.[105,106] If antihypertensives are required, nicardipine and clevidipine are both considered acceptable titratable options (Category C).

Disability

There are several physiologic changes during pregnancy that alter the clinical impact of TBI. The seizure threshold is reduced during pregnancy.[105] Moreover, conditions such as preeclampsia and eclampsia may be intercurrent with trauma; mental status change associated with head trauma is worrisome for traumatic intracranial hemorrhage, but preeclampsia and eclampsia must be considered.[13] When indicated, levetiracetam (Category C) is an acceptable antiepileptic in pregnant patients.[107]

Intracranial hypertension should be avoided in pregnant patients just as in nonpregnant patients. The definition of elevated ICP is not different in pregnancy; intracranial hypertension should be diagnosed for any sustained ICP greater than 20 mm Hg and cerebral perfusion pressure should be maintained at 50 to 60 mm Hg.[105] Just as in nonpregnant patients, several standard measures should be taken as first line to avoid intracranial hypertension; this includes raising the head of bed 30°, avoiding hypotension and hypertension, hyperthermia, hyperglycemia, hypoxia, anemia, and hyponatremia, and maintaining normocapnia.

The medical management of elevated ICPs in pregnancy remains somewhat of a black box; mannitol use has been reported in cases of intracranial hypertension secondary to intracranial tumors, and lower doses (0.25–0.5 g/kg) seem safe.[105,108] Animal studies suggest that mannitol may cause fetal dehydration, bradycardia, and hypoxia.[109] Intrauterine hypertonic saline was previously used for second-trimester abortions, but intravenous hypertonic has not been shown to have a deleterious effect.[105] Hyperventilation and hypocarbia should be avoided if possible, as it may decrease blood flow to the placenta.[108] Barbiturates should be avoided if possible, even in cases of refractory intracranial hypertension.[105] Therapeutic hypothermia may be considered.[105]

Patients may be at a higher risk for venous thromboembolism (VTE) due to hypercoagulability in pregnancy and should be started on deep venous thrombosis (DVT) prophylaxis early in the absence of contraindications (such as an intracranial or other significant bleed).[103] Furthermore, TBI may cause a decline in maternal progesterone levels, increasing risk of preterm labor or spontaneous abortion.[103]

Traumatic Spinal Cord Injury

There are guidelines for the care and management of women with existing SCIs who later become pregnant,[110] but discussions of SCI during pregnancy are limited. Although rare, some women experience a relative osteoporosis during pregnancy, which has been reported to increase risk of spinal fractures even with minor trauma, such as ground-level falls.[111–113] Acute SCI during pregnancy has been associated with a high risk of miscarriage, particularly early in pregnancy, as well as fetal malformations.[114,115] The same has not been true of pregnancy after SCI.[115]

Airway, breathing, circulation

The initial evaluation of pregnant patients with suspected SCI does not differ from the usual approach.[116] Supportive measures, and particularly the avoidance of hypoxia, hypotension, and fever, are essential to maternal and fetal recovery.[114] Airway and breathing should be closely monitored, with a low threshold for intubation and mechanical ventilation, given the high risk of respiratory failure in SCI and the high oxygenation and relatively specific ventilation demands associated with pregnancy.[116] Disruption of the sympathetic chain may lead to neurogenic shock, characterized by vasodilation (warm skin) and often, though not always, a paradoxic bradycardia. Because SCI often coexists with other significant injuries, clinicians must be careful to attribute hypotension solely to neurogenic shock, particularly given that the diagnosis of acute blood loss in pregnancy is already made difficult by increased circulating blood volume.[116] Nonetheless, vasopressors or inotropic support may be required to address hypotension in the setting of neurogenic shock, after careful fluid (or blood) resuscitation.[116–118] Neurogenic shock has been associated with significant decreases in fetal perfusion.[116] It may last anywhere from 1 to 3 weeks.[116,119] In conjunction with neurogenic shock, patients with high SCI may experience varying degrees of autonomic dysreflexia, resulting in intermittent hypertension. In the pregnant patient, it is difficult but crucial to differentiate this from preeclampsia.[119]

Management after stabilization

SCI are traditionally diagnosed using MRI, rather than CT scan, which allows for direct visualization of the spinal cord. MRI has not been associated with adverse events during pregnancy.[13] ACOG recommends the use of gadolinium be limited due to conflicting evidence regarding impact on fetal outcomes[13]; gadolinium is not typically required for the diagnosis of acute traumatic SCI. Surgical management of vertebral fractures with resulting SCI during pregnancy has been described in case reports with good outcomes.[111] Given the hypercoagulable state associated with pregnancy, and the high risk of VTE in acute SCI, DVT prophylaxis with low-molecular weight heparin should be initiated as soon as is safe.[116] It should also be remembered that, dependent on the level and severity of the injury, SCI may prevent a pregnant patient from feeling contractions, and they may be unaware when labor has begun.[119]

CLINICS CARE POINTS

- Pregnancy may not be evident, and many pregnancies are discovered incidentally during trauma evaluation.
- Leftward uterine displacement can be applied to improve maternal cardiac output and may require designated personnel to maintain to stabilize the patient.
- Although optimal perimortem cesarean delivery is within 5 minutes of arrest, reports of neurointact fetal survival and maternal benefit exist beyond 15 minutes.
- Standard RSI techniques and medications can be used safely in pregnancy, but may be more difficult, and special attention should be paid to preoxygenation, positioning, and possible mucosal edema or bleeding.
- Owing to maternal diaphragm elevation, chest tubes should be place 1 to 2 ribs spaces high to avoid abdominal placement in gravid patients.

DISCLOSURE

Dr. J. Downing has no financial disclosures. Dr L. Sjeklocha has no financial disclosures.

REFERENCES

1. Hill CC, Pickinpaugh J. Trauma and Surgical Emergencies in the Obstetric Patient. Surg Clin North Am 2008;88(2):421–40.

2. El-Kady D, Gilbert WM, Anderson J, et al. Trauma during pregnancy: an analysis of maternal and fetal outcomes in a large population. Am J Obstet Gynecol 2004;190(6):1661–8.

3. Fildes J, Reed L, Jones N, et al. Trauma: the leading cause of maternal death. J Trauma 1992;32(5):643–5.

4. World Health Organization. Global status report on road safety 2018. World Health Organization; 2018. Available at: https://apps.who.int/iris/handle/10665/276462. Accessed June 18, 2022.

5. Petrone P, Jiménez-Morillas P, Axelrad A, et al. Traumatic injuries to the pregnant patient: a critical literature review. Eur J Trauma Emerg Surg 2019;45(3):383–92.

6. Ford K, Menchine M, Burner E, et al. Leadership and teamwork in trauma and resuscitation. West J Emerg Med 2016;17(5):549–56.

7. Smith JA, Sosulski A, Eskander R, et al. Implementation of a multidisciplinary perinatal emergency response team improves time to definitive obstetrical evaluation and fetal assessment. J Trauma Acute Care Surg 2020;88(5):615–8.

8. American College of Surgeons, Committee on Trauma. Advanced trauma life support: student course manual.; 2018.

9. Jain V, Chari R, Maslovitz S, et al. Guidelines for the management of a pregnant trauma patient. J Obstet Gynaecol Can 2015;37(6):553–71.

10. Barraco RD, Chiu WC, Clancy TV, et al. Practice management guidelines for the diagnosis and management of injury in the pregnant patient: the east practice management guidelines work group. J Trauma Inj Infect Crit Care 2010;69(1):211–4.

11. Trauma during pregnancy. ACOG Technical Bulletin Number 161–November 1991. Int J Gynaecol Obstet Off Organ Int Fed Gynaecol Obstet 1993;40(2):165–70.

12. Petrone P, Marini CP. Trauma in pregnant patients. Curr Probl Surg 2015;52(8):330–51.

13. Jain C. ACOG committee opinion no. 723: guidelines for diagnostic imaging during pregnancy and lactation. Obstet Gynecol 2019;133(1):186.

14. Bochicchio GV, Napolitano LM, Haan J, et al. Incidental Pregnancy in Trauma Patients. J Am Coll Surg 2001;192(5):4.

15. Weiss HB. The epidemiology of traumatic injury-related fetal mortality in Pennsylvania, 1995–1997: the role of motor vehicle crashes. Accid Anal Prev 2001;33(4):449–54.

16. Roemer K, Beccera O, Bowes R. Trauma in the Obstetric Patient: A Bedside Tool. Available at: www.acep.org/by-medical-focus/trauma/trauma-in-the-obstetric-patient-a-bedside-tool/. Accessed July 1, 2022.

17. Mendez-Figueroa H, Dahlke JD, Vrees RA, et al. Trauma in pregnancy: an updated systematic review. Am J Obstet Gynecol 2013;209(1):1–10.

18. Drexler KA, Quist-Nelson J, Weil AB. Intimate partner violence and trauma-informed care in pregnancy. Am J Obstet Gynecol MFM 2022;4(2):100542.

19. Kuo C, Jamieson DJ, McPheeters ML, et al. Injury hospitalizations of pregnant women in the United States, 2002. Am J Obstet Gynecol 2007;196(2):161.e1–6.

20. Petrone P, Talving P, Browder T, et al. Abdominal injuries in pregnancy: a 155-month study at two level 1 trauma centers. Injury 2011;42(1):47–9.

21. Fischer PE, Zarzaur BL, Fabian TC, et al. Minor trauma is an unrecognized contributor to poor fetal outcomes: a population-based study of 78,552 pregnancies. J Trauma Inj Infect Crit Care 2011;71(1):90–3.

22. MacArthur B, Foley M, Gray K, et al. Trauma in pregnancy: a comprehensive approach to the mother and fetus. Am J Obstet Gynecol 2019;220(5):465–8.e1.

23. Tan EK, Tan EL. Alterations in physiology and anatomy during pregnancy. Best Pract Res Clin Obstet Gynaecol 2013;27(6):791–802.
24. Pilkington S, Carli F, Dakin MJ, et al. Increase in Mallampati score during pregnancy. Br J Anaesth 1995;74(6):638–42.
25. Mushambi MC, Kinsella SM, Popat M, et al. Obstetric Anaesthetists' Association and Difficult Airway Society guidelines for the management of difficult and failed tracheal intubation in obstetrics. Anaesthesia 2015;70(11):1286–306.
26. Lentz S, Grossman A, Koyfman A, et al. High-risk airway management in the emergency department: diseases and approaches, Part II. J Emerg Med 2020;59(4):573–85.
27. Kinsella SM, Winton AL, Mushambi MC, et al. Failed tracheal intubation during obstetric general anaesthesia: a literature review. Int J Obstet Anesth 2015; 24(4):356–74.
28. Pollard R, Wagner M, Grichnik K, et al. Prevalence of difficult intubation and failed intubation in a diverse obstetric community-based population. Curr Med Res Opin 2017;33(12):2167–71.
29. Einav S, Sela HY, Weiniger CF. Management and Outcomes of Trauma During Pregnancy. Anesthesiol Clin 2013;31(1):141–56.
30. Hegewald MJ, Crapo RO. Respiratory physiology in pregnancy. Clin Chest Med 2011;32(1):1–13.
31. Hignett R, Fernando R, McGlennan A, et al. A randomized crossover study to determine the effect of a 30° head-up versus a supine position on the functional residual capacity of term parturients. Anesth Analg 2011;113(5):1098–102.
32. Hill CC, Pickinpaugh J. Physiologic Changes in Pregnancy. Surg Clin North Am 2008;88(2):391–401.
33. Yeomans ER, Gilstrap LC. Physiologic changes in pregnancy and their impact on critical care. Crit Care Med 2005;33(Supplement):S256–8.
34. Brown S, Mozurkewich E. Trauma during pregnancy. Obstet Gynecol Clin North Am 2013;40(1):47–57.
35. LoMauro A, Aliverti A. Respiratory physiology of pregnancy: physiology masterclass. Breathe 2015;11(4):297–301.
36. LoMauro A, Aliverti A, Frykholm P, et al. Adaptation of lung, chest wall, and respiratory muscles during pregnancy: preparing for birth. J Appl Physiol 2019; 127(6):1640–50.
37. Di Napoli M, DeVoe WB, Leon S, et al. Decreased incidence of rib fractures in pregnant patients after motor vehicle collisions. Am J Crit Care 2021;30(5): 385–90.
38. Lapinsky SE. Management of acute respiratory failure in pregnancy. Semin Respir Crit Care Med 2017;38(2):201–7.
39. Jain V, Chari R, Maslovitz S, et al. Guidelines for the management of a pregnant trauma patient. J Obstet Gynaecol Can 2015;37(6):553–74.
40. Sanghavi M, Rutherford JD. Cardiovascular Physiology of Pregnancy. Circulation 2014;130(12):1003–8.
41. Clark SL, Cotton DB, Pivarnik JM, et al. Position change and central hemodynamic profile during normal third-trimester pregnancy and post partum. Am J Obstet Gynecol 1991;164(3):883–7.
42. Jeejeebhoy FM, Zelop CM, Lipman S, et al. Cardiac Arrest in Pregnancy: A Scientific Statement From the American Heart Association. Circulation 2015; 132(18):1747–73.
43. Spinella PC, Holcomb JB. Resuscitation and transfusion principles for traumatic hemorrhagic shock. Blood Rev 2009;23(6):231–40.

44. Holcomb JB, Tilley BC, Baraniuk S, et al. Transfusion of plasma, platelets, and red blood cells in a 1:1:1 vs a 1:1:2 ratio and mortality in patients with severe trauma: the PROPPR randomized clinical trial. JAMA 2015;313(5):471–82.
45. Buchsbaum HJ. Diagnosis and management of abdominal gunshot wounds during pregnancy. J Trauma 1975;15(5):425–30.
46. Raza SS, Tyler K, Najjar RJ. resuscitative endovascular balloon occlusion of the aorta in the management of a gunshot wound and rupture of the uterus. Am Surg 2022;88(4):784–6.
47. Khalifa A, Avraham JB, Kramer KZ, et al. Surviving traumatic cardiac arrest: Identification of factors associated with survival. Am J Emerg Med 2021; 43:83–7.
48. Teeter W, Haase D. Updates in traumatic cardiac arrest. Emerg Med Clin North Am 2020;38(4):891–901.
49. Lott C, Truhlář A, Alfonzo A, et al. European Resuscitation Council Guidelines 2021: Cardiac arrest in special circumstances. Resuscitation 2021;161: 152–219.
50. Moore EE, Knudson MM, Burlew CC, et al. Defining the limits of resuscitative emergency department thoracotomy: a contemporary western trauma association perspective. J Trauma Inj Infect Crit Care 2011;70(2):334–9.
51. Seamon MJ, Haut ER, Van Arendonk K, et al. An evidence-based approach to patient selection for emergency department thoracotomy: A practice management guideline from the Eastern Association for the Surgery of Trauma. J Trauma Acute Care Surg 2015;79(1):159–73.
52. Monsieurs KG, Nolan JP, Bossaert LL, et al. European Resuscitation Council Guidelines for Resuscitation 2015. Resuscitation 2015;95:1–80.
53. Soar J, Becker LB, Berg KM, et al. Cardiopulmonary resuscitation in special circumstances. The Lancet 2021;398(10307):1257–68.
54. On behalf of the SOS-KANTO 2012 Study Group, Yamamoto R, Suzuki M, Hayashida K, et al. Epinephrine during resuscitation of traumatic cardiac arrest and increased mortality: a post hoc analysis of prospective observational study. Scand J Trauma Resusc Emerg Med 2019;27(1):74.
55. Wongtanasarasin W, Thepchinda T, Kasirawat C, et al. Treatment Outcomes of Epinephrine for Traumatic Out-of-hospital Cardiac Arrest: A Systematic Review and Meta-analysis. J Emerg Trauma Shock 2021;14(4):195–200.
56. Healy ME, Kozubal DE, Horn AE, et al. Care of the Critically Ill Pregnant Patient and Perimortem Cesarean Delivery in the Emergency Department. J Emerg Med 2016;51(2):172–7.
57. Bickley LS, Szilagyi PG, Hoffman RM, et al. Bates' guide to physical examination and history taking. 13th edition. Philadelphia, USA: Wolters Kluwer; 2021.
58. Gatti F, Spagnoli M, Zerbi SM, et al. Out-of-hospital perimortem cesarean section as resuscitative hysterotomy in maternal posttraumatic cardiac arrest. Case Rep Emerg Med 2014;2014:1–4.
59. Drukker L, Hants Y, Sharon E, et al. Perimortem cesarean section for maternal and fetal salvage: concise review and protocol. Acta Obstet Gynecol Scand 2014;93(10):965–72.
60. Beckett V, Knight M, Sharpe P. The CAPS Study: incidence, management and outcomes of cardiac arrest in pregnancy in the UK: a prospective, descriptive study. BJOG Int J Obstet Gynaecol 2017;124(9):1374–81.
61. Katz V, Balderston K, DeFreest M. Perimortem cesarean delivery: Were our assumptions correct? Am J Obstet Gynecol 2005;192(6):1916–20.

62. Einav S, Kaufman N, Sela HY. Maternal cardiac arrest and perimortem caesarean delivery: Evidence or expert-based? Resuscitation 2012;83(10): 1191–200.
63. Ng WM, Lee WF, Cheah SO, et al. Peri-mortem caesarean section after traumatic arrest: Crisis resource management. Am J Emerg Med 2018;36(12): 2338.e1–3.
64. Singh S, Chawla S, Venigalla SK. Peri mortem cesarean section-when every second counts. Trends Anaesth Crit Care 2021;41:34–6.
65. Curry N, Brohi K. Surgery in traumatic injury and perioperative considerations. Semin Thromb Hemost 2020;46(01):073–82.
66. Huls CK, Detlefs C. Trauma in pregnancy. Semin Perinatol 2018;42(1):13–20.
67. Muench MV, Baschat AA, Reddy UM, et al. Kleihauer-betke testing is important in all cases of maternal trauma. J Trauma 2004;57(5):1094–8.
68. Soskin PN, Yu J. Resuscitation of the Pregnant Patient. Emerg Med Clin North Am 2019;37(2):351–63.
69. Matsunaga S, Takai Y, Seki H. Fibrinogen for the management of critical obstetric hemorrhage. J Obstet Gynaecol Res 2019;45(1):13–21.
70. Kush ML, Muench MV, Harman CR, et al. Persistent fetal hemoglobin in maternal circulation complicating the diagnosis of fetomaternal hemorrhage. Obstet Gynecol 2005;105(4):872–4.
71. Greco PS, Day LJ, Pearlman MD. Guidance for evaluation and management of blunt abdominal trauma in pregnancy. Obstet Gynecol 2019;134(6):1343–57.
72. Trivedi N, Ylagan M, Moore TR, et al. Predicting adverse outcomes following trauma in pregnancy. J Reprod Med 2012;57(1–2):3–8.
73. Muench MV, Baschat AA, Dorio PJ, et al. Successful pregnancy outcome after splenic artery embolization for blunt maternal trauma. J Trauma 2004;56(5): 1146–8.
74. Richards JR, Ormsby EL, Romo MV, et al. Blunt abdominal injury in the pregnant patient: detection with US. Radiology 2004;233(2):463–70.
75. Glantz C, Purnell L. Clinical utility of sonography in the diagnosis and treatment of placental abruption. J Ultrasound Med Off J Am Inst Ultrasound Med 2002; 21(8):837–40.
76. Tremblay E, Thérasse E, Thomassin-Naggara I, et al. Quality initiatives: guidelines for use of medical imaging during pregnancy and lactation. Radiogr Rev Publ Radiol Soc N Am Inc 2012;32(3):897–911.
77. American College of Radiology. ACR–SPR practice parameter for imaging pregnant or potentially pregnant adolescents and women with ionizing radiation. Resolution 39. 2014. Available at: http://www.acr.org/~/media/9e2ed55531fc4b4fa53ef3b6d3b25df8.pdf. Accessed June 29, 2022.
78. Marsh RM, Silosky M. Patient Shielding in Diagnostic Imaging: Discontinuing a Legacy Practice. AJR Am J Roentgenol 2019;212(4):755–7.
79. Begano D, Söderberg M, Bolejko A. To use or not use patient shielding on pregnant women undergoing ct pulmonary angiography: a phantom study. Radiat Prot Dosimetry 2020;189(4):458–65.
80. Committee Opinion No. 718. Update on immunization and pregnancy: tetanus, diphtheria, and pertussis vaccination. Obstet Gynecol 2017;130(3):e153–7.
81. Elkomy MH, Sultan P, Drover DR, et al. Pharmacokinetics of prophylactic cefazolin in parturients undergoing cesarean delivery. Antimicrob Agents Chemother 2014;58(6):3504–13.

82. Ragunathan K, Thorn J. Management of grade V splenic injury with splenic artery embolization in pregnancy: A case report. Case Rep Womens Health 2022; 34:e00391.

83. Athiel Y, Vivanti A, Tranchart H. Splenic embolization for abdominal trauma during pregnancy. J Visc Surg 2020;157(1):71–2.

84. Browns K, Bhat R, Jonasson O, et al. Thoracoabdominal gunshot wound with survival of a 36-week fetus. JAMA 1977;237(22):2409–10.

85. Sakala EP, Kort DD. Management of stab wounds to the pregnant uterus: a case report and a review of the literature. Obstet Gynecol Surv 1988;43(6):319–24.

86. Franger AL, Buchsbaum HJ, Peaceman AM. Abdominal gunshot wounds in pregnancy. Am J Obstet Gynecol 1989;160(5 Pt 1):1124–8.

87. Morris JA, Rosenbower TJ, Jurkovich GJ, et al. Infant survival after cesarean section for trauma. Ann Surg 1996;223(5):481–8 [discussion: 488-491].

88. Molina GA, Aguayo WG, Cevallos JM, et al. Prenatal gunshot wound, a rare cause of maternal and fetus trauma, a case report. Int J Surg Case Rep 2019;59:201–4.

89. Wei SH, Helmy M, Cohen AJ. CT evaluation of placental abruption in pregnant trauma patients. Emerg Radiol 2009;16(5):365–73.

90. Dijkerman ML, Breederveld-Walters ML, Pijpe A, et al. Management and outcome of burn injuries during pregnancy: A systematic review and presentation of a comprehensive guideline. Burns J Int Soc Burn Inj 2022; S0305-4179(22):00069.

91. Maghsoudi H, Samnia R, Garadaghi A, et al. Burns in pregnancy. Burns J Int Soc Burn Inj 2006;32(2):246–50.

92. Pacheco LD, Gei AF, VanHook JW, et al. Burns in pregnancy. Obstet Gynecol 2005;106(5 Pt 2):1210–2.

93. Guo SS, Greenspoon JS, Kahn AM. Management of burn injuries during pregnancy. Burns J Int Soc Burn Inj 2001;27(4):394–7.

94. Friedman P, Guo XM, Stiller RJ, et al. Carbon Monoxide Exposure During Pregnancy. Obstet Gynecol Surv 2015;70(11):705–12.

95. Longo LD, Hill EP. Carbon monoxide uptake and elimination in fetal and maternal sheep. Am J Physiol 1977;232(3):H324–30.

96. Elkharrat D, Raphael JC, Korach JM, et al. Acute carbon monoxide intoxication and hyperbaric oxygen in pregnancy. Intensive Care Med 1991;17(5):289–92.

97. Prasanna M, Singh K. Early burn wound excision in "major' burns with "pregnancy': a preliminary report. Burns J Int Soc Burn Inj 1996;22(3):234–7.

98. Koren G, Florescu A, Costei AM, et al. Nonsteroidal antiinflammatory drugs during third trimester and the risk of premature closure of the ductus arteriosus: a meta-analysis. Ann Pharmacother 2006;40(5):824–9.

99. U.S. Food & Drug Administration. FDA recommends avoiding use of NSAIDs in pregnancy at 20 weeks of later because they can result in low amniotic fluid. Published online October 15, 2020.

100. Griggs C, Goverman J, Bittner EA, et al. Sedation and pain management in burn patients. Clin Plast Surg 2017;44(3):535–40.

101. Roy AB, Hughes LP, West LA, et al. Meeting the challenge of analgesia in a pregnant woman with burn injury using subanesthetic ketamine: a case report and literature review. J Burn Care Res Off Publ Am Burn Assoc 2020;41(4): 913–7.

102. Correia-Sá I, Marques M, Horta R, et al. Experience in Management of Burn Injury During Pregnancy in a Burn Unit. J Burn Care Res Off Publ Am Burn Assoc 2021;42(2):232–5.

103. Blaya MO, Raval AP, Bramlett HM. Traumatic brain injury in women across lifespan. Neurobiol Dis 2022;164:105613.
104. Berry C, Ley EJ, Mirocha J, et al. Do pregnant women have improved outcomes after traumatic brain injury? Am J Surg 2011;201(4):429–32.
105. Godoy DA, Robba C, Paiva WS, et al. Acute Intracranial Hypertension During Pregnancy: Special Considerations and Management Adjustments. Neurocrit Care 2022;36(1):302–16.
106. Lee A, Ngan Kee WD, Gin T. A quantitative, systematic review of randomized controlled trials of ephedrine versus phenylephrine for the management of hypotension during spinal anesthesia for cesarean delivery. Anesth Analg 2002; 94(4):920–6.
107. Koubeissi M. Levetiracetam: more evidence of safety in pregnancy. Epilepsy Curr 2013;13(6):279–81.
108. Bharti N, Kashyap L, Mohan VK. Anesthetic management of a parturient with cerebellopontine-angle meningioma. Int J Obstet Anesth 2002;11(3):219–21.
109. Basso A, Fernández A, Althabe O, et al. Passage of mannitol from mother to amniotic fluid and fetus. Obstet Gynecol 1977;49(5):628–31.
110. American College of Obstetricians and Gynecologists. ACOG Committee Opinion: Number 275, September 2002. Obstetric management of patients with spinal cord injuries. Obstet Gynecol 2002;100(3):625–7.
111. Lenarz CJ, Wittgen CM, Place HM. Management of a pregnant patient with a burst fracture causing neurologic injury. A case report. J Bone Joint Surg Am 2009;91(7):1747–9.
112. Sarikaya S, Ozdolap S, Açikgöz G, et al. Pregnancy-associated osteoporosis with vertebral fractures and scoliosis. Joint Bone Spine 2004;71(1):84–5.
113. Bayram S, Ozturk C, Sivrioglu K, et al. Kyphoplasty for pregnancy-associated osteoporotic vertebral fractures. Joint Bone Spine 2006;73(5):564–6.
114. Engel S, Ferrara G. Obstetric outcomes in women who sustained a spinal cord injury during pregnancy. Spinal Cord 2013;51(2):170–1.
115. Göller H, Paeslack V. Pregnancy damage and birth-complications in the children of paraplegic women. Paraplegia 1972;10(3):213–7.
116. Kang AH. Traumatic spinal cord injury. Clin Obstet Gynecol 2005;48(1):67–72.
117. Baranović S, Maldini B, Cengić T, et al. Anesthetic management of acute cervical spinal cord injury in pregnancy. Acta Clin Croat 2014;53(1):98–101.
118. Gilson GJ, Miller AC, Clevenger FW, et al. Acute spinal cord injury and neurogenic shock in pregnancy. Obstet Gynecol Surv 1995;50(7):556–60.
119. Popov I, Ngambu F, Mantel G, et al. Acute spinal cord injury in pregnancy: an illustrative case and literature review. J Obstet Gynaecol J Inst Obstet Gynaecol 2003;23(6):596–8.

Cardiovascular Complications of Pregnancy

John Mark Sawyer, MD[a],*, Naseem Moridzadeh, MD[b], Rebecca A. Bavolek, MD[a]

KEYWORDS

- Venous thromboembolism • Pulmonary embolism • Deep venous thrombosis
- Superficial venous thrombosis • Acute myocardial infarction
- Spontaneous coronary artery dissection • Peripartum cardiomyopathy
- Aortic dissection

KEY POINTS

- The risk of all types of venous thromboembolism increases in the procoagulant state of pregnancy. This risk increases throughout the duration of pregnancy and into the post-partum period. Low-molecular weight heparin is the preferred treatment in the setting of pregnancy.
- Pregnancy poses an increased risk for acute myocardial infarction and spontaneous coronary artery dissection. Treatment is similar between the two, with the exception of thrombolytics. Ideally, patients should undergo coronary angiography whenever possible.
- Peripartum cardiomyopathy is managed similarly to other forms of cardiomyopathy, including noninvasive ventilation strategies, diuretics, and afterload reduction with nitroglycerin.
- Aortic dissection is a relatively low incidence but high mortality occurrence in pregnancy. Again, the management is similar to that of the nonpregnant patient, with surgical management being the preferred modality for Type A dissections and medical management for Type B dissections.

INTRODUCTION

The physiologic and hormonal changes of pregnancy present significant stress to the cardiovascular system. Maternal cardiac output increases by 50% and circulating blood volume may increase by as much as 100% to support the gestating fetus. The hormonal changes of pregnancy also increase the risk of thrombotic events and vascular dissections. As maternal age increases in the United States, more women are coming into pregnancy with significant preexisting conditions that are brought into sharp focus by these physiologic stresses. The clinical importance of cardiovascular conditions is highlighted by the fact that cardiovascular conditions combined with cardiomyopathy

[a] UCLA Ronald Reagan, Olive View Emergency Medicine Residency, 1100 Glendon Avenue, Suite 1200, Los Angeles, CA 90024, USA; [b] NYU Langone Health, 570 First Avenue, New York, NY 10016, USA
* Corresponding author.
E-mail address: johnsawyer@mednet.ucla.edu

Emerg Med Clin N Am 41 (2023) 247–258
https://doi.org/10.1016/j.emc.2023.01.005
0733-8627/23/© 2023 Elsevier Inc. All rights reserved.
emed.theclinics.com

account for 26.5% of pregnancy-related deaths in the United States, making this the leading cause of such deaths.[1] This review—targeted toward the emergency clinician—encompasses the major cardiovascular disorders of pregnancy and highlights their specific diagnostic challenges and new developments in the field.

VENOUS THROMBOEMBOLISM IN PREGNANCY

For the emergency clinician, the diagnosis and management of venous thromboembolism (VTE) is the most frequently encountered cardiovascular complication of pregnancy. VTE includes superficial vein thrombosis (SVT), deep vein thrombosis (DVT), and pulmonary embolus (PE) with PE being the most challenging diagnosis given the concern for maternal and fetal exposure to ionizing radiation and differing society guidelines.[2–7] VTE complicates 1.2 per 1000 deliveries and risk increases throughout pregnancy and into the postpartum period. The postpartum period has a variable definition but the risk for VTE seems to peak in the first week, declining to the prepregnancy risk after 12 weeks.[8]

Superficial Vein Thrombosis

Although rarely the primary concern of the emergency clinician approaching a pregnant or postpartum patient, SVT may be found in the diagnostic workup of DVT. In this case, the emergency clinician must assess the risk for a subsequent thrombotic event or clot extension. Particular attention should be given to SVT above the knee, extensive SVT (>5 cm), and close proximity to the saphenofemoral junction (within 3 cm) as these are considered higher risk for a subsequent thrombotic event.[9–11] The American Society of Hematology recommends treatment with low-molecular weight heparin (LMWH) for all proven SVT in pregnant patients—this recommendation was based on studies in the nonpregnant population because there are no studies including pregnant patients.[12] The largest of these is the CALISTO (Comparison of ARIXTRA™ in lower LImb Superficial Thrombophlebitis with placebo) trial, a placebo-controlled trial that found an 85% reduction in subsequent symptomatic PE, symptomatic DVT, extension to the sapheno-femoral junction, or recurrence for patients treated for SVT.[13] Given that pregnancy itself is a risk factor for VTE, patients in this group are at higher risk for extension and subsequent PE/DVT and, therefore, should be considered for prophylactic or therapeutic anticoagulation.

Deep Vein Thrombosis

Presenting symptoms of DVT in pregnancy are similar to those found in the nonpregnant patient with leg pain and swelling as the predominant symptoms. Due to direct compression of pelvic veins, the left lower extremity is more often involved and iliac or femoral DVT has a much higher prevalence—approximately 80% of DVTs in pregnant patients are proximal compared with less than 20% of nonpregnant patients.[14,15] The primary approach to diagnosis remains compression ultrasound. For those patients with intermediate-to-high probability of disease with a negative or equivocal compression ultrasound, further imaging with either duplex ultrasonography or venography (CT or noncontrast MR) should be pursued. Alternatively, in the right clinical situation, consideration may be given to empiric treatment. For all patients, 3 to 7 day follow-up ultrasound is recommended.[4]

Pulmonary Embolism

Up to 1.5 per 100,000 maternal deaths are due to PE in the United States and Europe, making PE the leading cause of maternal death in the developed world. Most of these deaths (60%) occur in the postpartum period.[16] Delays in diagnosis and treatment, along with inadequate thromboprophylaxis contribute significantly to these deaths.[17]

Many of the key clinical features of PE are confounded by the physiologic changes of pregnancy including tachycardia, tachypnea, dyspnea, and edema. These signs and symptoms are also incorporated into decision rules, such as modified Well's score and revised Geneva score, that are often used to risk stratify nonpregnant patients for PE. Unfortunately, these decision rules have not been validated in pregnant patients and studies show they may miss a significant number of PEs even in low-risk groups, as discussed in the previous edition of this article.[18]

New Evidence for D-dimer in the Pregnant Patient

The D-dimer test is a frequently used part of the clinical evaluation of PE that obviates the need for radiologic studies because it has excellent negative predictive value in the nonpregnant population.[19] It represents one of several fibrin degradation products, which is increased in the serum in the presence of a thrombus. It has been an area of controversy in the pregnant population because this serum marker increases throughout pregnancy, creating concern for false positives.

A 2019 study by Van der Pol and colleagues evaluated the YEARS-adjusted D-dimer algorithm in the setting of pregnancy in a prospective multicenter trial in the Netherlands. This study included 498 pregnant patients who all received a D-dimer test. The algorithm suggests PE is unlikely and no imaging is necessary if the D-dimer is less than 1000 ng/mL and the patient does not meet any of the 3 YEARS criteria: clinical signs of DVT, hemoptysis, and PE as the most likely diagnosis. In patients who meet one or more YEARS criteria, it is suggested that PE is unlikely, and imaging is not necessary if the D-dimer is less than 500 ng/mL. Between both groups that did not receive imaging, there was 1 DVT found at 3-month follow-up. The overall VTE rate was low with 20 patients having proven VTE in the study. This approach reduced the need for imaging by 65% in the first trimester and 32% in the third trimester.[20]

This study was subsequently incorporated into a systematic review by Bellesini and colleagues and was the largest of the 4 studies included. This systematic review included 1194 women from 4 different studies with a low-to-intermediate pretest probability of PE. The negative predictive value of the D-dimer test in this study was 1.00 with a confidence interval of 0.99 to 1.00. There was significant heterogeneity between the included studies, and unfortunately, there were few women included in the highest-risk postpartum period.[19] Subsequently, the European Society of Cardiology in conjunction with the European Respiratory Society recommended D-dimer testing for patients with low-to-intermediate pretest probability of PE as a means to avoid unnecessary radiologic testing.[7] At this time, this recommendation has, to our knowledge, not been incorporated into any US society guidelines.

The authors of this review agree that a negative D-dimer, particularly in early pregnancy, is a reasonable rule-out test in a low-to-intermediate risk group. Since the last edition of Emergency Medicine Clinics on the topic, the 2 studies above are major new additions to this area, although further prospective studies are needed, particularly including postpartum patients.

Imaging for Pulmonary Embolism in Pregnancy

The diagnosis of PE in pregnancy, as in the nonpregnant population, depends on thoracic imaging using ionizing radiation. Divergent recommendations exist on the optimal approach to imaging for PE, which are outlined in **Table 1**.[2,4,7]

For the patient with lower extremity symptoms or signs of DVT, it is reasonable to start with ultrasound and proceed to thoracic imaging if negative. If positive, the

Table 1
Summary of international society guidelines on diagnosis of venous thromboembolism in pregnancy

	Use of Clinical Decision Rules (Well's Geneva)?	Use of D-dimer?	Ultrasound Before CTPA for V/Q Scan?	CTPA or V/Q?
American College of Obstetrics and Gynecology (US)	No	No	Unclear	Agree with ATS-STR
American Thoracic Society/Society of Thoracic Radiology (US)	No	No	Yes, if LE symptoms	CXR (Chest X-ray) then V/Q if normal. If abnormal, CTPA is reasonable
European Society of Cardiology	With D-dimer	Yes	Yes, if LE symptoms	CXR and then either CTPA or V/Q If CXR abnormal, CTPA
Royal College of Obstetrics and Gynecology (UK)	No	No	Yes, if LE symptoms	CXR and then either CTPA or V/Q If CXR abnormal, CTPA

patient may be initiated on an appropriate anticoagulant drug with a presumptive diagnosis of pulmonary embolism. A limited echocardiogram to assess for right heart strain may be a useful additional study to add to this approach, particularly if the patient is hemodynamically unstable and being considered for thrombolytic therapy.

Both CT pulmonary angiography (CTPA) and ventilation-perfusion scanning (V/Q) are reasonable tests for the diagnosis of PE in the pregnant patient.[3,21] V/Q scanning requires a chest radiograph that is normal before proceeding with the study. Traditionally, V/Q scanning has been thought to result in more fetal radiation exposure than CTPA—although this is somewhat unclear. The CTPA clearly results in more maternal radiation exposure, particularly to breast tissue, which is particularly sensitive in this highly proliferative stage of life. The radiation exposure of V/Q scanning can be reduced by deferring the ventilation portion if the patient has a normal perfusion scan because this would not be suggestive of PE.[3]

CTPA has the advantages of elucidating alternate diagnoses, providing information about right heart strain, and having a lower rate of "nondiagnostic" studies compared with V/Q scanning.[3,22] It is also more readily available at all hours of the day in many emergency departments. Interestingly, modern CTPA may actually be superior to conventional pulmonary angiography in the non-pregnant population according to the American College of Radiology.[3]

A reasonable approach would be to discuss the preferred diagnostic pathway with your local radiology department and to develop a standardized local protocol before encountering this emergency department patient.

Treatment

LMWH is the preferred treatment of VTE in pregnancy and postpartum because it does not cross the placenta and does not cross into breast milk. The American Society of Hematology guidelines recommend LMWH with either once daily or twice daily dosing. The patient should have close subspecialty follow-up because the increased volume of distribution associated with the normal hypervolemia of pregnancy may affect serum levels. For patients with severe renal dysfunction, unfractionated heparin is the preferred treatment.[12] For the patient who is peripartum or periprocedural, a heparin drip may be preferred due to the ability to stop the infusion with rapid return to normal clotting parameters.[4,7]

Rarely a patient with a severe heparin allergy may be encountered. Although there is little evidence in this area, treatment with fondaparinux is recommended.[4,7]

Warfarin is generally not recommended in the pregnant or postpartum patient because it has known teratogenic effects and crosses into breast milk. Direct oral anticoagulants (DOACs) including the factor Xa inhibitors and direct thrombin inhibitors are not recommended in pregnancy due to a lack of evidence on safety and efficacy.[4] In postpartum patients, evidence for safety of DOACs is also lacking and there is some evidence it may cross into breast milk.[12]

For patients with hemodynamic instability due to PE, treatment with thrombolytic therapy is recommended.[4,7,12,23] For patients with evidence of right heart strain but who have not developed hemodynamic instability, thrombolytic therapy is not recommended.[12] Finally, for the crashing pregnant patient with PE extracorporeal membrane oxygenation (ECMO), if available, may be considered as a risky but necessary intervention.

In any patient with confirmed or ongoing concern for VTE, multidisciplinary involvement and/or close follow-up should be obtained. Carefully selected patients with DVT may be candidates for outpatient treatment. Most patients with confirmed PE will be admitted for management.

ACUTE MYOCARDIAL INFARCTION

Acute myocardial infarction (AMI) complicates approximately 3 per 100,000 pregnancies worldwide. However, in the United States, AMI complicates nearly 5 per 100,000 pregnancies and is associated with a higher maternal mortality rate.[24] Pregnancy itself is an independent risk factor for myocardial infarction with a 3-fold to 4-fold increase in risk.[25] Pregnancy-specific conditions such as eclampsia and preeclampsia also increase the risk of subsequent AMI. With the increasing prevalence of cardiovascular comorbidities and advanced maternal age, this problem may only grow as a significant contributor to the increasing cardiovascular deaths associated with pregnancy. The overall mortality from AMI in pregnancy is around 5%.[24–26]

Due to the increasing physiologic stresses throughout pregnancy, it is unsurprising that the incidence of AMI, although reported in all stages, increases throughout the course of pregnancy, with the highest risk in the peripartum and postpartum periods.[24,25,27] Pregnant women experience anemia due to a relative hemodilution, which occurs in spite of increased red blood cell mass and in turn compromises myocardial oxygen delivery. Myocardial oxygen demand is also increased because of increased stroke volume and heart rate.

The clinical presentation of AMI in pregnancy and postpartum includes chest pain, dyspnea, nausea, vomiting, and diaphoresis. Unfortunately, as discussed previously, pregnant women experience exertional dyspnea and fatigue that may be difficult to differentiate as physiologic versus pathologic cardiac symptoms.

The diagnostic approach is the same as in the nonpregnant patient and hinges on electrocardiogram (EKG) changes and elevated serum markers. An EKG should be obtained and, if ST-elevation myocardial infarction (STEMI) criteria are present, an emergent cardiac catheterization will be necessary to elucidate the diagnosis. A troponin level may also be suggestive of AMI but there is the possibility of an elevated troponin without the presence of coronary disease in the setting of preeclampsia or gestational hypertension.[28] In the case of AMI found to be due to plaque rupture or thrombosis, percutaneous coronary intervention (PCI) remains the treatment of choice. However, a significant number of pregnancy-associated AMIs are due to spontaneous coronary artery dissection (SCAD), which may be managed differently, as outlined below. Aspirin, nitrates, beta-blockers, and heparin are all considered safe in pregnancy and may be part of the emergency department treatment of the pregnant patient with AMI. The caveat for heparin, that is discussed below, is that there is a high prevalence of SCAD in this population.

Spontaneous Coronary Artery Dissection

SCAD accounts for up to 43% of pregnant patients presenting with STEMI and seems to occur in 1.8 per 100,000 pregnancies, making it the most common cause of AMI in this population.[29,30] SCAD is thought to occur secondary to weakened vessel walls, which leads to either an intramural hematoma that ruptures or an intimal flap that propagates and forms a false lumen.[31] The hormonal changes of pregnancy and hemodynamic stress applied to the vasculature are thought to predispose to SCAD. Traditional risk factors for SCAD include advanced maternal age, smoking history, hypertension, and diabetes.[31] Nonetheless, SCAD in the setting of pregnancy has been reported in many patients without these traditional risk factors for coronary artery disease. When compared with nonpregnant patients with SCAD, it seems that pregnant patients present more critically ill with a higher incidence of STEMI, proximal dissection, multivessel involvement, decreased LV systolic function, and cardiogenic shock.[27,31] SCAD generally occurs in the left main or left anterior descending circulation.[27,31] Patients generally present with chest pain, and it most often occurs in late pregnancy or in the early postpartum period.[27] This diagnosis is made in the catheterization suite by the interventionalist but awareness of this clinical condition is important for the emergency clinician because there are significant changes in the approach to treating SCAD. Notable changes are outlined below.

- Glycoprotein IIb/IIIa inhibitors are not recommended because they may increase the risk of propagation and bleeding.[31]
- Thrombolytics are not recommended because they may also further increase the risk of propagation of the false lumen.[31] Therefore, given the high prevalence of SCAD in this population, these patients should be transferred to a center with cardiac catheterization, if possible.
- Although the diagnosis is made by conventional coronary angiography, subsequent PCI is often less desirable unless the patient has refractory symptoms, refractory arrhythmias, or cardiogenic shock.
- Coronary artery bypass grafting is also an option in some of these patients with a better short-term outcome than PCI but with higher longer term graft failure than CABG in non-SCAD patients.[31]

The American Heart Association recommends that patients found to have SCAD are preferentially treated medically with beta-blocker, long-term aspirin, short-term clopidogrel, and with the addition of a statin in patients with dyslipidemia.[32,33] The emergency clinician managing a pregnant patient meeting STEMI criteria will not know the underlying cause and, thus, should consider administering heparin and other antiplatelets in conjunction with cardiology recommendations.

PERIPARTUM CARDIOMYOPATHY

Peripartum cardiomyopathy (PPCM) is a consideration in any patient in the later stages of pregnancy or postpartum who presents with dyspnea. It was formerly called postpartum cardiomyopathy and included any patient who developed idiopathic systolic heart failure within 5 months of delivery. However, the definition has been expanded to include patients who present in the last month of pregnancy with systolic heart failure.[34] As with the other entities discussed in this article, the presentation is confounded by significant symptomatic overlap with the normal physiologic changes of pregnancy and with other important disorders such as preeclampsia. Cardiomyopathy is a significant cause of pregnancy-related mortality, accounting for approximately 11% of deaths.[1] For patients with PPCM, the mortality rate is up to 28% with a mean mortality of 16%. A significant number of these patients also have a diagnosis of preeclampsia (~30%).[35] The signs and symptoms of PPCM include dyspnea on exertion, orthopnea, paroxysmal nocturnal dyspnea, edema, pulmonary rales, elevated jugular venous pressure, and chest tightness among others. With severely depressed ejection fraction, these patients may present in cardiogenic shock or with thromboembolic complications. Delays in diagnosis result in worse outcomes.[34]

The diagnosis of PPCM is one of exclusion and so is unlikely to be made in the emergency department before the exclusion of alternate causes (CAD, preexisting cardiac disease, hypertensive disorders of pregnancy, valvular disease, and so forth). The workup includes EKG, chest radiograph, troponin, and brain-natriuretic peptide. An echocardiogram will also be part of the workup and an emergency department bedside echocardiogram may be helpful in ruling in the diagnosis.

The management of PPCM is similar to that of heart failure in nonpregnant patients, including the use of noninvasive ventilation strategies, with a few exceptions.[28]

- During pregnancy, angiotensin converting enzyme (ACE) inhibitors, angiotensin receptor blockers and aldosterone antagonists are contraindicated.
- Diuretics may be initiated in patients with adequate SBP with the caveat that they may cause decreased placental blood flow.
- If afterload reduction is required, nitroprusside is contraindicated during pregnancy. However, the use of nitroglycerin is acceptable.
- Bromocriptine is an experimental treatment of patients with a previous diagnosis of PPCM.
- For patients with thromboembolic complications, heparin or LMWH is the preferred anticoagulation medication. Warfarin is contraindicated in pregnancy and breastfeeding.
- Early delivery through C-section may be indicated if the fetus is viable.

The principle of management for the critically ill pregnant patient remains supporting the hemodynamics of the mother because this is the most important factor influencing fetal survival. Norepinephrine and other vasopressors and inotropes are not thoroughly studied in pregnancy but should be used if necessary.[28] Other treatments such as mechanical circulatory support, ECMO, and implantable cardiac defibrillator (ICD) implantation may be indicated. Early involvement of obstetrics, cardiology, and critical care are paramount. Many women will ultimately have a full recovery but the course may be prolonged.

AORTIC DISSECTION

Pregnancy itself is thought to be an independent risk factor for aortic dissection, although this remains an extremely rare event, making definitive conclusions elusive.[36,37] The largest study of pregnancy-related aortic dissection included 44 total cases during a 20-year period, which accounted for 0.1% of all reported aortic dissections. Based on this, the resulting incidence of aortic dissection in all pregnancies is 0.0004%.[38] The increased cardiac output, due to both increased heart rate and stroke volume, produces more stress on the aortic walls allowing for the propagation of the dissection. Hormonal changes are thought to drive the histopathologic changes in the aortic intima and media that classically predispose to an intimal tear.[38–40] These vascular changes may actually persist for up to 12 months postpartum.[40] The most common risk factor identified for pregnancy-related aortic dissection seems to be preexisting aortopathy (Marfan syndrome, Loeys-Dietz syndrome, and other connective tissue disorders) or bicuspid aortic valve but most of these women are unfortunately unaware of their condition before pregnancy.[41] The incidence of aortic dissection, as with the other cardiovascular conditions covered in this article, seems to increase throughout pregnancy and peaks in the early postpartum period.[41]

Regarding the clinical presentation of aortic dissection in pregnancy, the most common presenting symptom remains chest pain, although it is not universally present.[42] Unfortunately, as with the nonpregnant patient, there is often a missed diagnosis or delay to diagnosis at initial presentation, which may be expected given the much higher incidence of alternate causes of chest pain.[43,44] Other presenting symptoms include syncope, nausea, vomiting, shortness of breath, and neurologic deficits. A delay to diagnosis is particularly concerning given the estimated hourly increase of 1% to 2% mortality. Although pregnancy-related changes confound the presentation, a detailed history and physical focusing on the quality of pain, radiation of pain, associated symptoms, new murmurs, and pulse differences are key to increasing the index of suspicion and ruling in the diagnosis.[45]

The diagnostic tests of choice for aortic dissection in the pregnant patient are the same as those in the nonpregnant patient. Due to widespread availability, high sensitivity, and high specificity, CT angiography of the aorta is the most commonly used test in the emergency department.[46] Trans-esophageal echocardiography (TEE) also has high sensitivity and specificity for thoracic aortic dissection and, if available, is a viable option that has the benefit of sparing exposure to radiation.[46] In an institution where cardiac anesthesiologists or cardiologists trained in TEE are in-house, consider requesting bedside TEE to confirm the diagnosis in unstable patients in the emergency department (ED) with thoracic aortic dissection. Finally, magnetic resonance (MR) aortography, while highly sensitive and specific, may not be useful in the pregnant patient. First, MR has limited availability in most hospitals, with the additional downside of taking a potentially unstable patient away from the emergency department for an extended period. Second, the most commonly available MR aorta protocols rely on administration of gadolinium contrast, which is contraindicated in pregnancy and relatively contraindicated in the breast-feeding mother.

Type A Stanford aortic dissection, involving the ascending aorta or arch, seems to account for ~67% of pregnancy-related aortic dissections.[47] As with the nonpregnant patient, early surgical consultation and intervention is key in the treatment of Type A aortic dissections. The surgical intervention of choice in later pregnancy is Caesarean section followed by immediate surgical repair of the aorta in the same operation.[44,47–49] Unfortunately, the maternal mortality seems to be up to 23%, whereas the fetal/neonatal mortality is 27% to 33%.[39,50]

For Type B Stanford aortic dissection, early surgical consultation is advised as well, although the need for surgical intervention depends on the clinical scenario. In both types of aortic dissection, emergency department management involves maternal cardiovascular control with vasoactive infusions, fetal heart rate monitoring, and early obstetric consultation. A heart rate goal of ~60 beats per minute should be targeted first using beta-blocker infusions, most commonly esmolol. After heart rate control has been achieved, afterload reduction with a goal systolic blood pressure (SBP) of less than 110 mm Hg should be targeted using calcium channel blocker infusion, most commonly nicardipine. It should be noted that ACE inhibitors and nitroprusside are contraindicated in pregnancy. For the patient that presents with shock, either due to acute aortic regurgitation, pericardial tamponade, or hemorrhage, a shift in focus to blood pressure support may be required.

CLINICS CARE POINTS

- When working up a pregnant patient for low-risk to intermediate probability VTE, applying the pregnancy-adjusted YEARS algorithm with D-dimer test is an emerging option that may reduce the need for further imaging.

- When evaluating a pregnant patient with STEMI, SCAD is a significant pathophysiologic mechanism in this population. Therefore, in the setting of STEMI in this population, routine administration of heparin is not recommended.

- The preferred anticoagulant in pregnancy, whether for VTE or other thrombotic complications, is heparin or LMWH. Warfarin is contraindicated in pregnancy, and DOACs are not well studied in pregnancy.

DISCLOSURES

None of the authors of this article has any commercial or financial conflicts of interest to disclose.

REFERENCES

1. Creanga AA, Syverson C, Seed K, et al. Pregnancy-Related Mortality in the United States, 2011-2013. Obstet Gynecol 2017;130(2):366–73.
2. Leung AN, Bull TM, Jaeschke R, et al. American Thoracic Society documents: an official American Thoracic Society/Society of Thoracic Radiology Clinical Practice Guideline–Evaluation of Suspected Pulmonary Embolism in Pregnancy. Radiology 2012;262(2):635–46.
3. Expert Panels on Cardiac and Thoracic I, Kirsch J, Brown RKJ, et al. ACR Appropriateness Criteria® Acute Chest Pain-Suspected Pulmonary Embolism. J Am Coll Radiol: JACR 2017;14(5S):S2–12.
4. American College of Obstetricians and Gynecologists' Committee on Practice BO. ACOG Practice Bulletin No. 196: Thromboembolism in Pregnancy. Obstet Gynecol 2018;132(1):e1–17.
5. American College of Emergency Physicians Clinical Policies Subcommittee on Thromboembolic D, Wolf SJ, Hahn SA, et al. Clinical Policy: Critical Issues in the Evaluation and Management of Adult Patients Presenting to the Emergency Department With Suspected Acute Venous Thromboembolic Disease. Ann Emerg Med 2018;71(5):e59–109.
6. Cohen SL, Feizullayeva C, McCandlish JA, et al. Comparison of international societal guidelines for the diagnosis of suspected pulmonary embolism during pregnancy. Lancet Haematology 2020;7(3):e247–58.
7. Konstantinides SV, Meyer G, Becattini C, et al. 2019 ESC Guidelines for the diagnosis and management of acute pulmonary embolism developed in collaboration with the European Respiratory Society (ERS). Eur Heart J 2020;41(4):543–603.
8. Heit JA, Kobbervig CE, James AH, et al. Trends in the incidence of venous thromboembolism during pregnancy or postpartum: a 30-year population-based study. Ann Intern Med 2005;143(10):697–706.
9. Galanaud JP, Bosson JL, Genty C, et al. Superficial vein thrombosis and recurrent venous thromboembolism: a pooled analysis of two observational studies. J Thromb Haemostasis: JTH 2012;10(6):1004–11.
10. Scovell SD, Ergul EA, Conrad MF. Medical management of acute superficial vein thrombosis of the saphenous vein. Journal of Vascular Surgery Venous and Lymphatic Disorders 2018;6(1):109–17.
11. Stevens SM, Woller SC, Baumann Kreuziger L, et al. Executive Summary: Antithrombotic Therapy for VTE Disease: Second Update of the CHEST Guideline and Expert Panel Report. Chest 2021;160(6):2247–59.
12. Bates SM, Rajasekhar A, Middeldorp S, et al. American Society of Hematology 2018 guidelines for management of venous thromboembolism: venous thromboembolism in the context of pregnancy. Blood Advances 2018;2(22):3317–59.
13. Decousus H, Prandoni P, Mismetti P, et al. Fondaparinux for the treatment of superficial-vein thrombosis in the legs. N Engl J Med 2010;363(13):1222–32.
14. Chan W-S, Spencer FA, Ginsberg JS. Anatomic distribution of deep vein thrombosis in pregnancy. CMAJ (Can Med Assoc J): Canadian Medical Association journal 2010;182(7):657–60.
15. Bukhari S, Fatima S, Barakat AF, et al. Venous thromboembolism during pregnancy and postpartum period. Eur J Intern Med 2022;97:8–17.

16. Abe K, Kuklina EV, Hooper WC, et al. Venous thromboembolism as a cause of severe maternal morbidity and mortality in the United States. Semin Perinatol 2019; 43(4):200–4.
17. Marik PE, Plante LA. Venous thromboembolic disease and pregnancy. N Engl J Med 2008;359(19):2025–33.
18. Borhart J, Palmer J. Cardiovascular Emergencies in Pregnancy. Emerg Med Clin 2019;37(2):339–50.
19. Bellesini M, Robert-Ebadi H, Combescure C, et al. D-dimer to rule out venous thromboembolism during pregnancy: A systematic review and meta-analysis. J Thromb Haemostasis 2021;19(10):2454–67.
20. van der Pol LM, Tromeur C, Bistervels IM, et al. Pregnancy-Adapted YEARS Algorithm for Diagnosis of Suspected Pulmonary Embolism. N Engl J Med 2019; 380(12):1139–49.
21. van Mens TE, Scheres LJ, de Jong PG, et al. Imaging for the exclusion of pulmonary embolism in pregnancy. Cochrane Database Syst Rev 2017;1:CD011053.
22. Sadeghi S, Arabi Z, Moradi M, et al. Diagnostic imaging to investigate pulmonary embolism in pregnancy using CT-Pulmonary angiography versus perfusion scan. J Res Med Sci 2021;26:37.
23. Martillotti G, Boehlen F, Robert-Ebadi H, et al. Treatment options for severe pulmonary embolism during pregnancy and the postpartum period: a systematic review. J Thromb Haemostasis 2017;15(10):1942–50.
24. Gibson P, Narous M, Firoz T, et al. Incidence of myocardial infarction in pregnancy: a systematic review and meta-analysis of population-based studies. European Heart Journal Quality of Care & Clinical Outcomes 2017;3(3):198–207.
25. James AH, Jamison MG, Biswas MS, et al. Acute myocardial infarction in pregnancy: a United States population-based study. Circulation 2006;113(12): 1564–71.
26. Ladner HE, Danielsen B, Gilbert WM. Acute myocardial infarction in pregnancy and the puerperium: a population-based study. Obstet Gynecol 2005;105(3): 480–4.
27. Tweet MS, Hayes SN, Codsi E, et al. Spontaneous Coronary Artery Dissection Associated With Pregnancy. J Am Coll Cardiol 2017;70(4):426–35.
28. Bauersachs J, König T, van der Meer P, et al. Pathophysiology, diagnosis and management of peripartum cardiomyopathy: a position statement from the Heart Failure Association of the European Society of Cardiology Study Group on peripartum cardiomyopathy. Eur J Heart Fail 2019;21(7):827–43.
29. Elkayam U, Jalnapurkar S, Barakkat MN, et al. Pregnancy-associated acute myocardial infarction: a review of contemporary experience in 150 cases between 2006 and 2011. Circulation 2014;129(16):1695–702.
30. Faden MS, Bottega N, Benjamin A, et al. A nationwide evaluation of spontaneous coronary artery dissection in pregnancy and the puerperium. Heart. British Cardiac Society) 2016;102(24):1974–9.
31. Hayes SN, Kim ESH, Saw J, et al. Spontaneous Coronary Artery Dissection: Current State of the Science: A Scientific Statement From the American Heart Association. Circulation 2018;137(19):e523–57.
32. Saw J, Aymong E, Sedlak T, et al. Spontaneous coronary artery dissection: association with predisposing arteriopathies and precipitating stressors and cardiovascular outcomes. Circulation Cardiovascular Interventions 2014;7(5):645–55.
33. Saw J. Spontaneous coronary artery dissection. Can J Cardiol 2013;29(9): 1027–33.

34. Davis MB, Arany Z, McNamara DM, et al. Peripartum Cardiomyopathy: JACC State-of-the-Art Review. J Am Coll Cardiol 2020;75(2):207–21.
35. Asad ZUA, Maiwand M, Farah F, et al. Peripartum cardiomyopathy: A systematic review of the literature. Clin Cardiol 2018;41(5):693–7.
36. Nasiell J, Lindqvist PG. Aortic dissection in pregnancy: the incidence of a life-threatening disease. Eur J Obstet Gynecol Reprod Biol 2010;149(1):120–1.
37. Kamel H, Roman MJ, Pitcher A, et al. Pregnancy and the Risk of Aortic Dissection or Rupture: A Cohort-Crossover Analysis. Circulation 2016;134(7):527–33.
38. Sawlani N, Shroff A, Vidovich MI. Aortic dissection and mortality associated with pregnancy in the United States. J Am Coll Cardiol 2015;65(15):1600–1.
39. De Martino A, Morganti R, Falcetta G, et al. Acute aortic dissection and pregnancy: Review and meta-analysis of incidence, presentation, and pathologic substrates. J Card Surg 2019;34(12):1591–7.
40. Rommens KL, Sandhu HK, Miller CC, et al. In-hospital outcomes and long-term survival of women of childbearing age with aortic dissection. J Vasc Surg 2021;74(4):1135–42.e1.
41. Braverman AC, Mittauer E, Harris KM, et al. Clinical Features and Outcomes of Pregnancy-Related Acute Aortic Dissection. JAMA cardiology 2021;6(1):58–66.
42. Meng X, Han J, Wang L, et al. Aortic dissection during pregnancy and postpartum. J Card Surg 2021;36(7):2510–7.
43. Lameijer H, Crombach A. Aortic Dissection During Pregnancy or in the Postpartum Period: It All Starts With Clinical Recognition. Ann Thorac Surg 2018; 105(2):663.
44. Ch'ng SL, Cochrane AD, Goldstein J, et al. Stanford type a aortic dissection in pregnancy: a diagnostic and management challenge. Heart Lung Circ 2013; 22(1):12–8.
45. Rosman HS, Patel S, Borzak S, et al. Quality of history taking in patients with aortic dissection. Chest 1998;114(3):793–5.
46. Expert Panel on Cardiac I, Kicska GA, Hurwitz Koweek LM, et al. ACR Appropriateness Criteria® Suspected Acute Aortic Syndrome. J Am Coll Radiol: JACR 2021;18(11S):S474–81.
47. Aziz F, Penupolu S, Alok A, et al. Peripartum acute aortic dissection: A case report & review of literature. J Thorac Dis 2011;3(1):65–7.
48. Yam N, Lo CS-Y, Ho CK-L. Acute Aortic Dissection Associated With Pregnancy. Ann Thorac Surg 2015;100(4):1470.
49. Rimmer L, Heyward-Chaplin J, South M, et al. Acute aortic dissection during pregnancy: Trials and tribulations. J Card Surg 2021;36(5):1799–805.
50. Jha N, Jha AK, Chand Chauhan R, et al. Maternal and Fetal Outcome After Cardiac Operations During Pregnancy: A Meta-Analysis. Ann Thorac Surg 2018; 106(2):618–26.

Nonobstetric Surgical Emergencies in Pregnancy

Caitlin L. Oldenkamp, MD*, Kellie Kitamura, MD

KEYWORDS

- Acute abdomen in pregnancy • Abdominal imaging in pregnancy
- Surgery in pregnancy

KEY POINTS

- Physical examination of the abdomen is limited by the gravid uterus.
- Laboratory studies can mimic infection and anemia.
- Early surgical intervention leads to fewer maternal and neonatal complications.

INTRODUCTION

Abdominal pain is a common complaint during pregnancy with causes ranging from benign to acutely life-threatening conditions. Emergency physicians must avoid the temptation to cognitively anchor on obstetric causes of abdominal pain and maintain a high index of suspicion for acute, nonobstetric causes. This task is made all the more difficult by pregnancy-associated deviations in vital signs, laboratory results, and physical examination. Furthermore, emergency physicians must also consider the impact of imaging on the developing fetus.

Nonobstetric surgery occurs in 1 to 2 out of 1000 pregnancies with appendectomy and cholecystectomy being the first and second most common operations, respectively.[1] Delays to surgery are the greatest predictors of postoperative morbidity in pregnant patients, which makes imperative a thoughtful, thorough, and timely evaluation in the emergency department.[2]

EVALUATION IN THE EMERGENCY DEPARTMENT
History

Emergency physicians should generally approach acute abdominal pain in the pregnant patient in the same way as nonpregnant patients. Physicians should additionally obtain past and present obstetric history, including gestational age, access to prenatal

The authors have nothing to disclose.
UCLA Ronald Reagan/Olive View Emergency Medicine Program, 924 Westwood Boulevard, Suite 300, Los Angeles, CA 90095, USA
* Corresponding author.
E-mail address: coldenkamp@mednet.ucla.edu

Emerg Med Clin N Am 41 (2023) 259–267
https://doi.org/10.1016/j.emc.2023.01.001
0733-8627/23/© 2023 Elsevier Inc. All rights reserved.
emed.theclinics.com

care, history of bleeding disorders, prior episodes of pregnancy-associated abdominal pain, and past delivery complications.

Nausea and vomiting are common complaints during the first trimester of pregnancy but are less commonly attributable to obstetric causes during the second and third trimesters. After 20 weeks of gestation, nausea and vomiting require further workup, especially when co-occurring with fever, focal abdominal pain, or vital sign derangements. Abdominal pain that is accompanied by vaginal leaking or bleeding often points to an obstetric cause. Evaluation of pregnant trauma victims is discussed in a separate and dedicated section.

Examination

The abdominal examination in pregnant patients becomes progressively limited by the expanding uterus. The gravid uterus extends from the pelvis into the abdominal cavity at approximately 12 weeks of gestation.[3] Abdominal organs translate cranially within the abdominal cavity to accommodate the expanding uterus in the following weeks. This organ displacement can cause atypical abdominal examinations for otherwise typical abdominal disease and may delay the development and recognition of peritoneal signs. Serial abdominal examinations may be warranted.

Continuous fetal heart rate monitoring is indicated in all patients with a viable pregnancy (approximately 22 weeks of gestation and greater). Fetal distress may occur secondary to maternal distress from both obstetric and nonobstetric causes. Signs of fetal distress may indicate the need for urgent delivery.

Laboratories

Physiologic changes of pregnancy can create diagnostic uncertainty for the emergency physician. Laboratory values can mimic both infection and hemorrhage. Pregnancy can increase a patient's baseline white blood cell count to 14,000 cells/mm^3, which can be misinterpreted and may spuriously lead emergency physicians to overdiagnose an infection.[4,5] In addition, pregnancy can also cause a mild thrombocytopenia (100 $\times$ 10^9 cells/L).[6]

Throughout pregnancy, blood plasma volume increases disproportionately to erythrocyte mass, resulting in a relative hemodilution seen during the second and third trimesters. Mean corpuscular volume and mean corpuscular hemoglobin concentration typically remain unchanged, which in the appropriate clinical context could be misinterpreted as evidence of active bleeding.[4,7]

Clinical pearls

- *Abdominal examination is distorted in the second and third trimesters*
- *Baseline laboratory work in pregnancy can mimic sepsis or acute hemorrhage*
- *Obtain continuous fetal monitoring for gestational age of 22 weeks or greater*

IMAGING

Imaging is fundamental to the workup of acute abdominal pain but requires careful consideration within pregnant populations due to the effects of ionizing radiation on the developing fetus. Current data is derived from survivors of the Chernobyl accident and the atomic bombing of Hiroshima and Nagasaki.[8,9]

The developing fetus is most sensitive to ionizing radiation during the 8 weeks following conception. In the initial 14 days following conception (i.e., the preembryonic phase) radiation-exposed pregnancies exhibit an all-or-none phenomenon; either the pregnancy survives undamaged or is fully resorbed.[10] Organogenesis occurs in the following 6 weeks and exposure to ionizing radiation can cause profound congenital anomalies during this period and is best avoided if possible.

Ultrasonography

Bedside ultrasonography is both familiar and readily available to the emergency physician, allowing for rapid, radiation-free imaging of abdominopelvic organs. The Rapid Ultrasound for Shock and Hypotension (RUSH) protocol can be useful in narrowing the differential diagnosis in hemodynamically unstable patients. The RUSH protocol incorporates the ultrasonographic windows of the Focused Assessment with Sonography for Trauma (FAST) examination, allowing for the detection of intraperitoneal free fluid. Sensitivity of the FAST examination ranges from 78% to 100% and is similar in both pregnant and nonpregnant populations.[11–13]

Although ultrasonography is the preferred imaging modality in pregnancy, it may not be sufficient in the workup of acute abdominal pain. Ultrasound images may be limited by patient body habitus, operator skill, and limited viewing windows. In addition, the gravid uterus functions to impede ultrasound imaging by displacing abdominal organs and obstructing abdominal views.

X-ray and Computed Tomography

Plain films offer minimal radiation exposure but have limited utility in the workup of undifferentiated abdominal pain in the emergency department, with the exception of diagnosing intestinal obstruction or for the identification of free air.

Computed tomography (CT) is essential to the workup of acute abdominal pain in the emergency department because it offers rapid image acquisition, excellent spatial resolution, and consistent performance regardless of patient or operator factors. Despite its use of ionizing radiation, CT remains the first-line imaging modality in pregnant patients who are hemodynamically unstable or victims of trauma. The risk of missing a life-threatening surgical emergency vastly outweighs the risk of fetal radiation exposure, especially as fetal survival explicitly depends on maternal survival. For these reasons, absolute contraindications for CT do not exist for any trimester in pregnancy.[14]

Magnetic Resonance Imaging

MRI is an attractive alternative to CT because it offers cross-sectional imaging without exposing the fetus to ionizing radiation. Access to MRI in the emergency department, especially during nonbusiness hours can prove challenging and produce delays to time-sensitive diagnoses. Image acquisition can take 1 to 2 hours, which is impractical for acutely ill patients. In such cases, CT imaging may be preferred.

Contrast Agents

The use of contrast agents may be necessary in the workup of acute abdominal pain. Iodinated contrast agents are able to cross the placenta but can be safely used throughout gestation with only minimal sequelae. Fetal thyroid function may become transiently depressed from the contrast agent's iodine load but no teratogenesis, carcinogenesis, or clinical sequelae have been observed.[15,16]

In contrast, gadolinium contrast agents are not recommended for use in pregnant patients due to their teratogenicity in animal models.[17] Human data shows in utero gadolinium exposure increases fetal risk for rheumatologic, inflammatory, or infiltrative skin conditions in addition to stillbirths and neonatal death.[18]

Clinical pearls

- *FAST examination has similar sensitivity in pregnant and nonpregnant patients*
- *CT scan is the imaging modality of choice in unstable pregnant patients*
- *MRI can be used as an alternative to CT but should not delay diagnosis*
- *Iodinated contrast agents are safe to use. Avoid gadolinium.*

DIFFERENTIAL DIAGNOSIS
Appendicitis

Acute appendicitis is the most common cause of surgery in pregnancy, occurring in approximately 1 per 1000 pregnancies.[19,20]

Classical history for acute appendicitis includes migratory abdominal pain, anorexia, nausea, vomiting, and fever. Examination historically includes tenderness over McBurney point in the right lower quadrant. These typical presentations of acute appendicitis are more likely to occur in early pregnancy, before distortion of the abdominal organs by the gravid uterus. During late pregnancy, in the second and third trimesters, patients may present atypically, with more vague and less focal abdominal pain. Physical examination may not demonstrate tenderness over McBurney point because the appendix may translate cranially toward the right upper quadrant.

First-line imaging is ultrasonography; however, its sensitivity in pregnant populations varies from 67% to 100% and up to 88% of studies are deemed nondiagnostic.[21–23] Second-line imaging in pregnancy is either MRI or CT of the abdomen, depending on institutional availability. Delays to diagnosis are associated with increased surgical complications and worse clinical outcomes for both mother and fetus.[24]

Emergency department management includes fluid resuscitation, initiation of antibiotics, and surgical consultation. Appendectomy is standard in pregnant populations but case report data suggests intravenous antibiotic therapy alone may be a successful treatment option if surgical services cannot be obtained in a timely manner.[25] Postoperative complication rates are similar between pregnant and nonpregnant patients undergoing laparoscopic appendectomy.[26]

Gallstone Disease

Pregnancy's hormonal milieu creates a favorable environment for gallstone formation with approximately 8% of all pregnant patients forming new gallstones by their third trimester.[27] Increased estrogen levels promote cholesterol secretion and increased progesterone levels cause gallbladder hypomotility and cholestasis, leading to high rates of gallstone formation.[28] Interestingly, prepregnancy obesity and multiparity each function as independent risk factors for the formation of gallstones during pregnancy.[29,30]

Pregnant patients with gallstone disease present with similar symptoms as their nonpregnant counterparts: nausea, vomiting, postprandial pain in the right upper quadrant and epigastrium. Positive Murphy sign is variably seen on physical examination.

Pregnancy alone increases alkaline phosphatase level, undermining its diagnostic utility. Liver enzymes and bilirubin, by contrast, do not typically increase during pregnancy; any abnormal elevations should prompt thorough investigation in the emergency department. Ultrasound, either bedside or formal, is the first-line imaging modality for suspected biliary disease.

Acute cholecystitis occurs in approximately 1 per 1600 pregnancies and cholecystectomy ranks as the second most common nonobstetric surgery performed during pregnancy.[31] Surgical management is favored over conservative, nonsurgical management due to fewer associated maternofetal complications (e.g., antepartum hemorrhage, amniotic fluid infection, preterm labor, preterm delivery, and abortion).[1,25,31,32]

Emergency department management includes fluid resuscitation, intravenous antibiotics if indicated, and surgical consultation. Other types of gallstone disease (i.e., choledocholithiasis, cholangitis, gallstone pancreatitis) are managed similarly between pregnant and nonpregnant patients and often require inpatient intervention with endoscopic retrograde cholangiopancreatography.

Aortic Dissection

Aortic dissection in pregnancy is rare but is often precipitated by either underlying connective tissue disorders or Turner syndrome. Patients with Marfan syndrome have the greatest risk (i.e., 3%) of pregnancy-associated aortic dissection.[33,34]

Survival of Stanford Type A (i.e., proximal to and including the great vessels of the aortic arch) dissections is time-dependent. Mortality rate is 1% to 3% per hour and increases to 30% within the initial 24 hours.[35] Alarmingly, median time-to-diagnosis can be delayed up to 18.5 hours in pregnant populations.[36]

Presentation most often consists of sudden-onset, migrating chest or back pain in addition to unequal radial pulses, gross hematuria, or neurological deficits.[37] D-dimer cannot be used to rule out low-risk dissection as pregnancy elevates baseline levels. CT angiography of the aorta is the first-line imaging modality in both pregnant and nonpregnant patients.

Management in the emergency department includes control of blood pressure and heart rate and immediate cardiothoracic surgery consultation.

Perforated Ulcer

Peptic ulcer disease (PUD) can be easily misdiagnosed as gastroesophageal reflux disease (GERD), which is common in pregnancy. PUD is far less benign than GERD and is the primary risk factor for gastrointestinal ulcer perforation.[38] Ulcer perforation classically presents as a triad of sudden-onset abdominal pain, tachycardia, and abdominal rigidity. Associated symptoms include diffuse abdominal pain, nausea, and vomiting.

Although plain films are often unhelpful in acute abdomen, they may be useful in evaluation of gastrointestinal ulcer perforation. Upright chest x-rays function to screen for subdiaphragmatic free air. Ultimately, the patient may still require cross-sectional imaging depending on their clinical presentation. Emergency interventions include fluid resuscitation, antibiotics that cover gastrointestinal flora, and prompt surgical consultation.

Hepatic Rupture

Spontaneous hepatic rupture is rare among pregnant patients, occurring in up to 1 per 45,000 to 225,000 deliveries.[39] The exact pathophysiology of spontaneous hepatic rupture in pregnancy is poorly understood but seems to be influenced by complications from preeclampsia and Hemolysis, Elevated Liver enzymes, Low Platelet count (HELLP) syndrome, including subcapsular hepatic hematoma formation.[39,40]

Hepatic rupture most often occurs during the third trimester and is highly lethal to both mother and fetus. Presentation includes hypotension and hemorrhagic shock in the setting of sudden-onset abdominal pain in the right upper quadrant and epigastrium. Pain may radiate to the back and shoulders.

Extrahepatic bleeding may be seen on ultrasound but stable patients will likely need cross-sectional imaging to confirm diagnosis.[41] Emergency physicians will need to trigger massive blood transfusion protocols. Fetal delivery is indicated following maternal stabilization and should be done in conjunction with surgical and obstetric teams.

Splenic Artery Aneurysm Rupture

Splenic artery aneurysms (SAAs) are typically asymptomatic unless they rupture. The hormonal and hemodynamic changes of pregnancy are thought to promote splenic artery aneurysm formation but their true prevalence is unknown.[42,43] Unfortunately, the same factors that promote SAA formation in pregnancy also promote SAA rupture, which most often occurs in the third trimester. SAA rupture is associated with maternal and fetal mortality rates up to 75% and 95%, respectively.[42]

Presentation may mimic a pulmonary embolism or placental abruption and often consists of sharp, abrupt-onset abdominal pain accompanied by hemodynamic collapse.[42,44] Bedside ultrasound may be used to quickly assess for free fluid in the peritoneum and prompt immediate surgery if positive. Confirmation of aneurysm rupture most often occurs by direct visualization in the operating room. Definitive treatment is ligation of the bleeding artery.

Mesenteric Venous Thrombosis

Mesenteric venous thrombosis (MVT) is a rare diagnosis in pregnancy but can lead to bowel ischemia, infarction, and perforation, if missed.[45] Pregnancy can increase the risk of MVT because it induces hypercoagulability and predisposes the mesenteric veins to compression from the expanding gravid uterus.

Presentation varies but can consist of nausea, vomiting, and poorly localized abdominal pain that is disproportionate to examination. CT angiography of the mesenteric vessels is the imaging of choice. Initial treatment is volume resuscitation, bowel rest, and anticoagulation.[46] Prompt surgical consultation is warranted given the high risk for bowel ischemia.

Intestinal Obstruction

Bowel obstruction is rare in pregnancy but the risk increases throughout gestation because abdominal organs shift to accommodate the gravid uterus. Approximately 25% of all bowel obstructions in pregnancy are attributable to colonic volvulus.[47] Additional risk factors for volvulus are abdominal adhesions, colonic enlargement, Hirschsprung disease, and intestinal malrotation.[48]

Signs and symptoms are similar between pregnant and nonpregnant patients: nausea, vomiting, obstipation, pain, and abdominal distention. Nausea and vomiting can be normal in the setting of early pregnancy but is uncommon and warrants clinical investigation once past 20 weeks of gestation.

Diagnosis is often made with cross-sectional imaging, although plain films and ultrasonography may be able to detect high-grade obstruction. Clinical management does not differ between stable pregnant and nonpregnant patients.

Adnexal Torsion

Adnexal torsion is estimated to account for 3% of female patients presenting with acute abdominal pain. Adnexal torsion can occur in any trimester of pregnancy but most commonly occurs during the first and is rare in the third. Traditional risk factors for adnexal torsion include ovarian mass or cyst. The risk of pregnancy-specific torsion is increased by participation in reproductive assistance technologies.[49]

Presentation usually consists of nausea, vomiting, and unilateral pelvic pain. Ultrasonography with Doppler is the imaging modality of choice to assess for adnexal torsion. Definitive diagnosis is made intraoperatively.[50] Viable ovaries are mechanically detorqued to restore blood flow. Necrotic and nonviable ovaries are surgically removed, which can affect future fertility.

SUMMARY

Abdominal pain in pregnancy must be thoroughly evaluated because many causes are time-sensitive and life-threatening to both the mother and fetus. Emergency physicians must maintain a high index of suspicion for both obstetric and nonobstetric causes of acute abdominal pain. Emergency physicians must also prepare to aggressively resuscitate unstable pregnant patients, which includes familiarity with resuscitative hysterotomy in the second and third trimesters.

CLINICS CARE POINTS

- Delays to diagnosis and surgical intervention increase maternofetal morbidity and mortality.
- Appendicitis and cholecysitis are common in pregnant populations.
- Ultrasound and MRI are preferable to CT imaging when available. CT imaging is preferred in unstable patients or when contrast is needed. Gadolinium is contraindicated in pregnant patients.
- Aggressive resuscitation may include resuscitative hysterotomy.

REFERENCES

1. Silvestri MT, Pettker CM, Brousseau EC, et al. Morbidity of appendectomy and cholecystectomy in pregnant and nonpregnant women. Obstet Gynecol 2011; 118(6):1261–70.
2. Gilo NB, Amini D, Landy HJ. Appendicitis and cholecystitis in pregnancy. Clin Obstet Gynecol 2009;52(4):586–96.
3. Walls RM, Hockberger RS, Gausche-Hill M, editors. Rosen's emergency medicine: concepts and clinical practice. 9th edition. Philadelphia, PA: Elsevier; 2018.
4. Soma-Pillay P, Nelson-Piercy C, Tolppanen H, et al. Physiological changes in pregnancy. Cardiovasc J Afr 2016;27(2):89–94.
5. Lurie S, Rahamim E, Piper I, et al. Total and differential leukocyte counts percentiles in normal pregnancy. Eur J Obstet Gynecol Reprod Biol 2008;136(1):16–9.
6. Practice ACOG. Bulletin no. 207: thrombocytopenia in pregnancy. Obstet Gynecol 2019;133(3):e181–93.
7. Kuklina EV, Ayala C, Callaghan WM. Hypertensive disorders and severe obstetric morbidity in the United States. Obstet Gynecol 2009;113(6):1299–306.
8. Otake M, Schull WJ, Yoshimaru H. A review of forty-five years study of Hiroshima and Nagasaki atomic bomb survivors. Brain damage among the prenatally exposed. J Radiat Res 1991;32(Suppl):249–64.
9. Wertelecki W. Malformations in a Chernobyl-impacted region. Pediatrics 2010; 125(4):e836–43.
10. De Santis M, Cesari E, Nobili E, et al. Radiation effects on development. Birth Defects Res C Embryo Today 2007;81(3):177–82.
11. Goodwin H, Holmes JF, Wisner DH. Abdominal ultrasound examination in pregnant blunt trauma patients. J Trauma 2001;50(4):689–94.

12. Brenchley J, Walker A, Sloan JP, et al. Evaluation of focused assessment with sonography in trauma (FAST) by UK emergency physicians. Emerg Med J 2006; 23(6):446–8.

13. Adams B, Sisson C. Review: bedside ultrasonography has 82% sensitivity and 99% specificity for blunt intraabdominal injury. Ann Intern Med 2012;157(4):2–12.

14. Lie G, Eleti S, Chan D, Roshen M, Cross S, Qureshi M. Imaging the acute abdomen in pregnancy: a radiological decision-making tool and the role of MRI. Clin Radiol 2022;77(9):639–49.

15. Raymond J, LaFranchi SH. Fetal and neonatal thyroid function: review and summary of significant new findings. Curr Opin Endocrinol Diabetes Obes 2010; 17(1):1–7.

16. Rajaram S, Exley CE, Fairlie F, et al. Effect of antenatal iodinated contrast agent on neonatal thyroid function. Br J Radiol 2012;85(1015):e238–42.

17. Chen MM, Coakley FV, Kaimal A, et al. Guidelines for computed tomography and magnetic resonance imaging use during pregnancy and lactation. Obstet Gynecol 2008;112(2):333–40.

18. Ray JG, Vermeulen MJ, Bharatha A, et al. Association between mri exposure during pregnancy and fetal and childhood outcomes. JAMA 2016;316(9):952–61.

19. Abbasi N, Patenaude V, Abenhaim HA. Management and outcomes of acute appendicitis in pregnancy-population-based study of over 7000 cases. BJOG 2014;121(12):1509–14.

20. Andersen B, Nielsen TF. Appendicitis in pregnancy: diagnosis, management and complications. Acta Obstet Gynecol Scand 1999;78(9):758–62.

21. Segev L, Segev Y, Rayman S, et al. The diagnostic performance of ultrasound for acute appendicitis in pregnant and young nonpregnant women: a case-control study. Int J Surg 2016;34:81–5.

22. Williams R, Shaw J. Ultrasound scanning in the diagnosis of acute appendicitis in pregnancy. Emerg Med J 2007;24(5):359–60.

23. Freeland M, King E, Safcsak K, et al. Diagnosis of appendicitis in pregnancy. Am J Surg 2009;198(6):753–8.

24. Ashbrook M, Cheng V, Sandhu K, et al. Management of complicated appendicitis during pregnancy in the us. JAMA Netw Open 2022;5(4):e227555.

25. Carstens AK, Fensby L, Penninga L. Nonoperative treatment of appendicitis during pregnancy in a remote area. AJP Rep 2018;08(01):e37–8.

26. Seok JW, Son J, Jung KU, et al. Safety of appendectomy during pregnancy in the totally laparoscopic age. J Minim Invasive Surg 2021;24(2):68–75.

27. Celaj S, Kourkoumpetis T. Gallstones in pregnancy. JAMA 2021;325(23):2410.

28. Nasioudis D, Tsilimigras D, Economopoulos KP. Laparoscopic cholecystectomy during pregnancy: a systematic review of 590 patients. Int J Surg 2016;27: 165–75.

29. Igbinosa O, Poddar S, Pitchumoni C. Pregnancy associated pancreatitis revisited. Clin Res Hepatol Gastroenterol 2013;37(2):177–81.

30. Liu B, Beral V, Balkwill A. Million Women Study Collaborators. Childbearing, breastfeeding, other reproductive factors and the subsequent risk of hospitalization for gallbladder disease. Int J Epidemiol 2009;38(1):312–8.

31. Schwulst SJ, Son M. Management of gallstone disease during pregnancy. JAMA Surg 2020;155(12):1162–3.

32. Cheng V, Matsushima K, Sandhu K, et al. Surgical trends in the management of acute cholecystitis during pregnancy. Surg Endosc 2021;35(10):5752–9.

33. Beirer M, Banke IJ, Münzel D, et al. Emergency cesarean section due to acute aortic dissection type a (Debakey i) without marfan syndrome: a case report and review of the literature. J Emerg Med 2014;46(1):e13–7.
34. Lipscomb KJ, Smith JC, Clarke B, et al. Outcome of pregnancy in women with Marfan's syndrome. Br J Obstet Gynaecol 1997;104(2):201–6.
35. Vallée M, Pineault-Lepage J, Ouimet D, et al. A case of an aortic dissection in a young adult: a refresher of the literature of this "great masquerader". Int J Gen Med 2011;889.
36. Ch'ng SL, Cochrane AD, Goldstein J, et al. Stanford type A aortic dissection in pregnancy: a diagnostic and management challenge. Heart Lung Circ 2013; 22(1):12–8.
37. Mészáros I, Mórocz J, Szlávi J, et al. Epidemiology and clinicopathology of aortic dissection. Chest 2000;117(5):1271–8.
38. Essilfie P, Hussain M, Bolaji I. Perforated duodenal ulcer in pregnancy-a rare cause of acute abdominal pain in pregnancy: a case report and literature review. Case Rep Obstet Gynecol 2011;2011:263016.
39. Augustin G, Hadzic M, Juras J, et al. Hypertensive disorders in pregnancy complicated by liver rupture or hematoma: a systematic review of 391 reported cases. World J Emerg Surg 2022;17(1):40.
40. Nunes JO, Turner MA, Fulcher AS. Abdominal imaging features of HELLP syndrome: a 10-year retrospective review. AJR Am J Roentgenol 2005;185(5): 1205–10.
41. Barton JR, Sibai BM. Hepatic imaging in HELLP syndrome (Hemolysis, elevated liver enzymes, and low platelet count). Am J Obstet Gynecol 1996;174(6):1820–5 [discussion: 1825-1827].
42. Sadat U, Dar O, Walsh S, et al. Splenic artery aneurysms in pregnancy–a systematic review. Int J Surg 2008;6(3):261–5.
43. Selo-Ojeme DO, Welch CC. Review: Spontaneous rupture of splenic artery aneurysm in pregnancy. Eur J Obstet Gynecol Reprod Biol 2003;109(2):124–7.
44. Richardson AJ, Bahlool S, Knight J. Ruptured splenic artery aneurysm in pregnancy presenting in a manner similar to pulmonary embolus. Anaesthesia 2006;61(2):187–9.
45. Atakan Al R, Borekci B, Ozturk G, et al. Acute mesenteric venous thrombosis due to protein S deficiency in a pregnant woman. J Obstet Gynaecol Res 2009;35(4): 804–7.
46. Salim S, Zarrouk M, Elf J, et al. Improved prognosis and low failure rate with anticoagulation as first-line therapy in mesenteric venous thrombosis. World J Surg 2018;42(11):3803–11.
47. Chase DM, Sparks DA, Dawood MY, et al. Cecal Volvulus in a Multiple-Gestation Pregnancy. Obstet Gynecol 2009;114(2):475–7.
48. Le CK, Nahirniak P, Anand S, et al. Volvulus. [Updated 2022 Sep 12]. In: StatPearls [Internet]. Treasure Island (FL): StatPearls Publishing; 2022 Jan-. Available from: https://www.ncbi.nlm.nih.gov/books/NBK441836/
49. Smorgick N, Pansky M, Feingold M, et al. The clinical characteristics and sonographic findings of maternal ovarian torsion in pregnancy. Fertil Steril 2009;92(6): 1983–7.
50. Melcer Y, Maymon R, Pekar-Zlotin M, et al. Does she have adnexal torsion? Prediction of adnexal torsion in reproductive age women. Arch Gynecol Obstet 2018; 297(3):685–90.

Hypertensive Disorders of Pregnancy

Nathaniel Coggins, MD*, Steven Lai, MD

KEYWORDS

• Gestational hypertension • Preeclampsia • Eclampsia • HELLP syndrome

KEY POINTS

- Hypertensive disorders in pregnancy are the second leading cause of global maternal and fetal morbidity and affect 5% to 10% of all pregnancies in the United States.
- The four hypertensive disorders of pregnancy include chronic hypertension, gestational hypertension, preeclampsia-eclampsia, and chronic hypertension with superimposed preeclampsia.
- A lower threshold for initiation of antihypertensive medication is recommended in pregnant patients with non-severe range gestational hypertension or preeclampsia without severe features or end-organ damage.
- Intravenous magnesium is the first-line treatment for patients with preeclampsia with severe features or eclampsia.
- First-line antihypertensive medications for acute management of severe range hypertension include labetalol, hydralazine, and nifedipine.

INTRODUCTION

Hypertensive disorders in pregnancy are the second leading cause of global maternal and fetal morbidity[1] and affect 5% to 10% of all pregnancies in the United States.[2,3] Even elevated systolic blood pressures (SBPs) below the diagnostic limit are associated with preterm delivery, small gestational weight, and low birth weight;[4,5] therefore, early recognition and initiation of appropriate therapies in the emergency department is critical to protecting the health of the mother and fetus.[6] Traditionally, hypertension in pregnancy has been defined as a blood pressure >140/90 mm Hg; however, there is variability in recommendations regarding when to initiate antihypertensive medication during pregnancy due to uncertainty about maternal benefits, medication effects on uteroplacental circulation, and medication effects on fetal development due to direct exposure. In recent years, there have been minor changes to the American College of Obstetrics and Gynecology (ACOG) and American College of Cardiology (ACC)/

UCLA-Olive View Emergency Medicine Program, 924 Westwood Boulevard, Suite 300, Los Angeles, CA 90095, USA
* Corresponding author.
E-mail address: ncoggins@mednet.ucla.edu

Emerg Med Clin N Am 41 (2023) 269–280
https://doi.org/10.1016/j.emc.2023.01.002
0733-8627/23/© 2023 Elsevier Inc. All rights reserved.
emed.theclinics.com

American Heart Association (AHA) guidelines for diagnosis and treatment of hypertension. This article reviews the different types of disorders of hypertension in pregnancy and how to diagnose and manage these patients, with special attention paid to any recent changes made to this management algorithm.

Classification of Hypertensive Disorders of Pregnancy

The four types of hypertensive disorders in pregnancy are chronic hypertension, gestational hypertension, preeclampsia-eclampsia, and chronic hypertension with superimposed preeclampsia.

Chronic Hypertension

In 2017, the ACC/AHA task force redefined hypertension for all adults as stage 1 hypertension if the SBP is > 130 mm Hg or the diastolic blood pressure (DBP) is > 80 mm Hg, and stage 2 hypertension if the SBP >140 mm Hg or the DBP is > 90 mm Hg. This change was made to address data that reflected modifiable long-term cardiovascular risk in stage 1 hypertension ranges.[7] The effect of ACC/AHA changes in women of reproductive age and on pregnancy outcomes is unknown, and as of 2019, ACOG still recognizes the traditional diagnostic cutoffs of SBP >140 mm Hg or DBP >90 mm Hg measured twice at least 4 hours apart.

Chronic hypertension during pregnancy is defined as hypertension diagnosed before pregnancy, before 20 weeks gestational age, or hypertension diagnosed during pregnancy that lasts >12 weeks following pregnancy. In contrast, gestational hypertension is defined as hypertension diagnosed after 20 weeks of gestational age. For women who present after 20 weeks without known prepregnancy blood pressure values, the differentiation between chronic hypertension and gestational hypertension can be challenging. Previously undiagnosed hypertension may be masked by pregnancy-related physiologic decreases in systemic vascular resistance in the first and second trimesters, with a return to prepregnancy levels by the third trimester. This can lead to mislabeling of chronic hypertension as gestational hypertension or preeclampsia.

Chronic hypertension can be divided into two categories based on underlying pathophysiology: primary and secondary hypertension. Primary hypertension is hypertension without any known underlying cause and accounts for approximately 86% of women with hypertension predating pregnancy.[8] Secondary hypertension accounts for less than 14%, and can be caused by underlying renal disease, vascular disease, or endocrinopathies.[8]

Chronic hypertension is further classified according to severity, with an increased risk of maternal and fetal complications as hypertension becomes more severe. Mild-to-moderate hypertension is defined as SBP 140 to 159 mm Hg or DBP 99 to 109 mm Hg, and severe hypertension is defined as SBP >160 mm Hg or DBP >110 mm Hg. Up to 20% to 50% of women with any degree of chronic hypertension and up to 78% of women with severe chronic hypertension may develop superimposed preeclampsia.[9–12] Women with uncomplicated chronic hypertension also have higher rates of gestational diabetes, indicated preterm delivery and planned c-section before labor, and postpartum hemorrhage. The fetal effects of chronic hypertension are fetal growth restriction and perinatal mortality, with rates of perinatal mortality two to four times higher than that of the general population.[13]

Gestational Hypertension

Gestational hypertension, often referred to as transient or pregnancy-induced hypertension, is defined as an SBP >140 mm Hg or DBP >90 mm Hg that develops after

20 weeks of gestational age and resolves within 12 weeks after delivery.[14,15] If blood pressures remain elevated 12 weeks after delivery, the diagnosis is changed to chronic hypertension. Risk factors for gestational hypertension include age less than 20 years and older than 40 years, obesity, hyperlipidemia, preexisting diabetes, African American race, family history of gestational hypertension, and nulliparity.[16–19]

Gestational hypertension is further classified according to severity, with severe gestational hypertension defined as an SBP $\geq$160 mm Hg, or a DBP $\geq$110 mm Hg, or both.[20] This distinction is important, as both maternal and perinatal outcomes for patients with severe gestational hypertension are significantly worse. More specifically, women with severe gestational hypertension have higher rates of preterm delivery and delivery of small-for-gestational-age infants 10. Similarly, women with severe gestational hypertension have higher rates of rare, severe maternal complications, such as acute kidney injury, thrombocytopenia, microangiopathic hemolysis, and hepatocellular necrosis.[21]

Patients with gestational hypertension are generally asymptomatic; however, all patients who meet the criteria for gestational hypertension should be initially screened for preeclampsia and other evidence of end-organ damage. This screening should include a careful history, review of systems, physical examination, urinalysis, blood analysis, and tocodynamometry, if appropriate. Among patients diagnosed with gestational hypertension, up to 50% will develop preeclampsia, with higher rates of progression to preeclampsia when diagnosed with gestational hypertension before 32 weeks.[22–24] Given this high rate of progression, all patients diagnosed with gestational hypertension should have a urinalysis, platelet counts, and liver enzymes evaluated weekly.[20] The differentiation between gestational hypertension and preeclampsia, however, does not appear to have many pragmatic implications, as the management is similar for gestational hypertension and preeclampsia without severe features.

Preeclampsia-Eclampsia

Preeclampsia is defined as new onset hypertension diagnosed after 20 weeks gestation with SBP >140 mm Hg or DBP >90 mm Hg with proteinuria or end-organ damage.[20] Preeclampsia is sometimes categorized as late onset if diagnosed after 34 weeks of gestation, as there is evidence that late-onset preeclampsia has a higher incidence of perinatal death and severe neonatal morbidity.[25] Although classically defined as new hypertension with concurrent proteinuria, the diagnostic criteria were expanded in 2013, and now include gestational hypertension in the absence of proteinuria with concurrent thrombocytopenia, abnormal liver function tests, epigastric or right upper quadrant pain with no alternative etiology, acute kidney injury, pulmonary edema, visual disturbances, or new-onset headache unresponsive to acetaminophen.[20,26–28] The presence of lower extremity edema should raise suspicion for preeclampsia; however, it is not included in the diagnostic criteria due to its prevalence in normal pregnancy.[29] Any patient diagnosed with gestational hypertension who has evidence of end-organ damage as outlined above should be diagnosed with preeclampsia. Furthermore, any patient diagnosed with severe range gestational hypertension who has evidence of end-organ damage as outlined above should be diagnosed with preeclampsia with severe features.

Hemolysis, elevated liver enzymes, and low platelets (HELLP) syndrome is a severe form of preeclampsia, and can lead to decreased placental perfusion and increased fetal and maternal morbidity and mortality.[30] HELLP syndrome occurs in 5% to 10% of patients with preeclampsia and is characterized by microangiopathic hemolytic anemia and thrombocytopenia.[31] Patients with HELLP syndrome most commonly present with right upper quadrant pain, malaise, nausea, and vomiting.[32,33] As a variant of preeclampsia with severe features, it is not uncommon for patients with HELLP syndrome to present with symptoms of preeclampsia with severe features, including headache, pulmonary edema, and vision changes. HELLP syndrome can present atypically, with up to 15% of patients presenting without hypertension or proteinuria 20. Although diagnosed primarily in the third trimester, up to 30% of cases are diagnosed after delivery, so postpartum follow-up and repeat blood analysis for individuals with preeclampsia with and without severe features is recommended.[20]

Eclampsia is defined as a generalized tonic-clonic, focal, or multifocal seizure in a preeclamptic patient without another underlying cause. Eclamptic seizures are usually tonic-clonic, lasting 60 to 90 s, and followed by a post-ictal phase.[34] In most of the cases, eclampsia is preceded by signs of cerebral irritation, including severe headaches, blurry vision, photophobia, and altered mental status. However, eclampsia can also occur without warning signs.[35,36] The terms preeclampsia and eclampsia suggest a natural progression from preeclampsia to eclampsia; however, approximately 38% of patients have abrupt onset of eclamptic seizures without a prior diagnosis of hypertension or proteinuria.[35] Eclampsia most commonly occurs antepartum or intrapartum, with most of the cases occurring after 28 weeks gestation. However, up to one-third of eclampsia-induced seizures occur postpartum, with the vast majority of those occurring within 48 hours of delivery.[37,38] Eclampsia can cause severe maternal hypoxia, traumatic injury associated with loss of consciousness, aspiration pneumonia, and both fetal and maternal death.[20] Eclampsia is associated with a maternal mortality rate of up to 14% and a fetal mortality rate of up to 1% worldwide.[39,40]

Both preeclampsia and eclampsia are associated with posterior reversible encephalopathy syndrome (PRES). PRES is defined as MRI evidence of vasogenic edema and hyperintensities in the posterior aspect of the brain. Patients at the highest risk for PRES have preeclampsia or eclampsia with concurrent headache, vision changes, or altered mental status.[41] Although neurologic deficits in the setting of preeclampsia and eclampsia are typically reversible, persistent deficits have been reported.[42]

Chronic Hypertension with Superimposed Preeclampsia

Chronic hypertension with superimposed preeclampsia is defined as preeclampsia in the setting of hypertension diagnosed before pregnancy or before 20 weeks gestation. Superimposed preeclampsia complicates approximately 50% of pregnant patients with chronic hypertension.[9,11,43] Risk factors for superimposed preeclampsia include African American race, obesity, history of tobacco use, longstanding hypertension (4 years or more), diastolic blood pressure greater than 100 mm Hg, or history of preeclampsia. There is no tool for predicting who will develop superimposed preeclampsia, and the diagnosis can be difficult to make. In general, patients with chronic hypertension develop preeclampsia earlier in their pregnancy and will present with a sudden increase in their baseline hypertension or proteinuria or develop new thrombocytopenia or elevated liver enzymes. This diagnosis is important to make, as patients with chronic hypertension with superimposed preeclampsia have worse maternal and fetal complications than patients with either chronic hypertension or preeclampsia alone.[9,44]

DIAGNOSIS

Hypertensive disorders of pregnancy should be considered in any pregnant patient who is found to have an SBP >140 mm Hg or DBP >90 mm Hg. The diagnosis of hypertensive disorders of pregnancy begins with determining when the hypertension started. More specifically, it is important to determine if the elevated blood pressure predates 20 weeks gestational age or developed at or after 20 weeks of gestation. Given changes made by the ACC/AHA, there are now more women that carry the diagnosis of stage 1 hypertension at time of pregnancy. Although ACOG still recognizes the traditional numerical cut-offs for hypertension, they state that it is reasonable to continue managing these patients as chronically hypertensive. In cases where no pre-pregnancy blood pressures are available for reference, ACOG recommends a higher degree of observation for women who have blood pressures in stage 1 hypertension ranges, as there is some data to suggest a higher risk of preeclampsia, gestational diabetes, and indicated preterm birth in this patient population.[45]

A careful history should be obtained to evaluate for the presence of any severe features, including headache, vision changes, shortness of breath, abdominal pain, and peripheral edema. Risk factors should be reviewed, including age, BMI, comorbidities, parity, race, family history, and history of hypertensive disorders of pregnancy. The patient should be assessed for physical examination correlates of severe features, including changes to visual acuity, retinal examination to assess for retinal hemorrhages, retinal edema, or papilledema, abdominal tenderness, crackles consistent with pulmonary edema, worsening peripheral edema, and hyperreflexia. It is important to note that benign peripheral edema is common during pregnancy; however, clinicians should have a high suspicion of preeclampsia-eclampsia if there is an abrupt change in the severity of peripheral edema.

All patients with an SBP >140 mm Hg or DBP >90 mm Hg, or symptoms and examination findings consistent with preeclampsia with severe features should have laboratory analysis performed. Laboratory analysis should include a complete blood count, basic metabolic panel, liver function tests, lactate dehydrogenase (LDH), uric acid, and urinalysis. More specifically patients should be evaluated for proteinuria ($\geq$300 mg/dL of protein in a 24-h urine collection or a protein-to-creatinine ratio $\geq$0.30), thrombocytopenia (platelet count <100 $\times$ 10^9/L) abnormal liver function tests (twice the upper limit of normal serum concentrations), acute kidney injury (serum creatinine concentration >1.1 mg/dL or a doubling of the serum creatinine concentration in the absence of another cause), or inappropriate rise in uric acid. Uric acid is an inconsistent predictor for preeclampsia, therefore its utility is debated; however, an inappropriate rise in uric acid should raise concern for preeclampsia in the right clinical setting.[46–48] If HELLP syndrome is suspected, an LDH level should be obtained to help identify hemolysis. HELLP syndrome is diagnosed by elevated LDH ($\geq$600 IU/L), elevated liver functions tests (twice the upper limit of normal serum concentrations), and thrombocytopenia (platelet count <100 $\times$ 10^9/L).[20,30,31]

PREVENTION
Aspirin

Low-dose aspirin can help prevent preeclampsia in patients at high risk. High risk is defined as a patient with (a) one high-risk factor, including the history of preeclampsia, chronic hypertension, multifetal gestation, renal disease, autoimmune disease, or diabetes, or (b) two moderate risk factors, including nulliparity, maternal age $\geq$35 years, obesity, family history of preeclampsia, and specific sociodemographic or personal history factors.[20] All women at high risk for preeclampsia should ideally be started on aspirin 81 mg/d between 12 to 16 weeks of gestation, though low-dose aspirin can be started as late as 28 weeks of gestation.[49,50] Low-dose aspirin should be continued until delivery.

Magnesium

Magnesium infusion can help prevent the progression of preeclampsia to eclampsia.[51] All preeclamptic patients with severe features or evidence of impending eclampsia should receive magnesium. A loading dose of magnesium is 4 to 6 g intravenously (IV) over 20 to 30 min followed by an infusion of 1 to 2 g/h 51. The administration of magnesium alone can reduce the incidence of the seizure by over 50% and has been shown to be superior to both benzodiazepines and phenytoin.[51–53] Magnesium toxicity can occur, therefore respiratory rate and blood pressure should be checked every 30 min, urine output checked every hour, and reflexes checked after administration of the loading dose and every 2 hours thereafter.[20] If the patient develops respiratory depression or hyporeflexia, 1 g of calcium gluconate can be administered intravenously to reverse the effects. The maintenance rate should be titrated to these findings, not serum magnesium concentration. The evidence does not support the routine use of magnesium prophylaxis in preeclampsia without severe features.[54]

MANAGEMENT
Antihypertensive Therapy

When presented with a hypertensive pregnant patient in the emergency department, it is important that the provider identify the disease process, presence of severe features, and initiate treatment to minimize symptoms and help prevent progression to eclampsia. There is consensus that all pregnant patients with severe range hypertension (SBP $\geq$160 mm Hg or DBP $\geq$110 mm Hg) confirmed by a repeat blood pressure measurement within 15 min should be started on an antihypertensive agent. It has been shown that prompt treatment within 30 to 60 min or as soon as reasonably possible can prevent serious fetal and maternal complications.[20,55,56]

There is less consensus regarding the treatment of non-severe hypertension in pregnant patients. Historically, pregnant patients who were found to have non-severe range gestational hypertension or preeclampsia without severe features or end-organ damage were referred for outpatient monitoring of blood pressure.[20] This practice guideline was based on several studies wherein treatment of non-severe range hypertension did not show a significant reduction in preeclampsia, perinatal death, preterm birth, or placental abruption.[55,57] This practice has been called into question by a recent study that showed a reduction in preeclampsia with severe features, preterm birth, abruption, and fetal or neonatal death with the treatment of non-severe range hypertension.[58] Given the results from this study, some organizations have recommended using SBP $\geq$140 mm Hg or DBP $\geq$90 mm Hg as the threshold for initiation of antihypertensive medication. The degree to which the blood pressure should be lowered is similarly debated, as there is mixed data regarding the blood pressure level below which there may be risk for placental hypoperfusion and growth restriction.[58,59]

First-line antihypertensive agents for the treatment of hypertensive disorders of pregnancy are labetalol, hydralazine, nifedipine, and methyldopa.[60,61] For the acute management of severe hypertension, intravenous labetalol, hydralazine, and oral immediate-release nifedipine can be used (**Table 1**).

Oral formulations of labetalol, hydralazine, and nifedipine can be used for ambulatory management of hypertensive disorders of pregnancy when delivery is not imminent. Methyldopa is a centrally-acting alpha-2 agonist that can also be used for the ambulatory management of hypertensive disorders of pregnancy. Methyldopa has a well-established fetal safety profile and can be a useful option for patients who cannot tolerate other oral antihypertensive medications.[56,62,63] It can be difficult to achieve adequate blood pressure control on methyldopa, and higher doses can cause sedation which may limit its use.

Table 1
Antihypertensive medication for acute management of preeclampsia with severe features or eclampsia

Drug	Mechanism	Dose	Considerations
Labetalol	Nonselective β-blocker	*Initial dose*: 5 to 10 mg IV over 2 min. *Repeat dose*: 20 to 80 mg IV every 10 min if SBP ≥ 160 mm Hg or DBP ≥ 110 mm Hg. Maintenance: 1 to 2 mg/min *Maximum dose*: 300 mg over 24 h.	*Side effects*: bronchospasm and bradycardia. Avoid in patients with a history of reactive airway disease, bradycardia, or any other contraindication to beta-blockade.
Hydralazine	Peripheral vasodilator	*Initial dose*: 5 to 10 mg IV over 2 min. *Repeat dose*: 10 mg IV every 20 min if SBP ≥ 160 mm Hg or DBP ≥ 110 mm Hg. *Maintenance*: 0.5 to 10 mg/min. *Maximum dose*: 20 to 30 mg over 24 h.	*Side effects*: headache, maternal hypotension, and reflex tachycardia. Avoid in patients with hemodynamic lability. Consider other agents if the heart rate is > 100 beats per minute after administration of 20 to 30 mg.
Nifedipine	Dihydropyridine calcium channel blocker	*Initial dose*: 10 mgPO. *Repeat dose*: 10 to 20 mg PO every 20 min if SBP ≥ 160 mm Hg or DBP ≥ 110 mm Hg. *Maximum dose*: 180 mg over 24 h.	*Side effects*: headache and reflex tachycardia. Consider carefully if the patient requires concurrent magnesium given the increased risk for hypotension (Ben-Ami et al.)

Ambulatory management at home should only be considered for patients with gestational hypertension or preeclampsia without severe features. If home management is selected, prompt follow-up with Obstetrics and Gynecology is recommended, as frequent fetal and maternal evaluations are required. Admission should be considered for patients with gestational hypertension or preeclampsia if blood pressure persists above 140/99 mm Hg, if the patient has severe features or end-organ damage, or if adherence to frequent monitoring is a concern.[20,30]

Delivery

The only definitive treatment for gestational hypertension, preeclampsia, or eclampsia is delivery; however, the timing of delivery must weigh the benefits of continued gestation against the risks of disease complications. If a patient presents with eclampsia, the acute management should prioritize stabilization, including a secure airway and initiation of a rapid-acting antihypertensive medication. If the fetus is between 24 to 34 weeks of gestational age, administration of betamethasone or dexamethasone is recommended to promote fetal lung maturity. Emergent consultation with an obstetrician should not be delayed, as delivery is indicated regardless of gestational age.[20]

If a patient has preeclampsia with severe features, delivery is recommended at 34 weeks of gestation once the patient has been stabilized. Delivery at 34 weeks helps avoid acute and long-term complications from preeclampsia. Furthermore, delivery should not be delayed for the administration of steroids.[20] If a patient is less than 34 weeks and is diagnosed with preeclampsia with severe features, expectant management can be considered; however, this decision should be made in conjunction with an obstetrician.

In patients without severe features, normal antepartum testing, and absence of preterm labor or premature rupture of membranes, continued monitoring until delivery at 37 weeks of gestation is recommended.

SUMMARY

Hypertensive disorders in pregnancy are a leading cause of global maternal and fetal morbidity. The four hypertensive disorders of pregnancy are chronic hypertension, gestational hypertension, preeclampsia-eclampsia, and chronic hypertension with superimposed preeclampsia. A careful history, review of systems, physical examination, and laboratory analysis can help differentiate these disorders and quantify the severity of the disease, which holds important implications for disease management.

CLINICS CARE POINTS

- Given recent recommendations by the American Heart Association/American College of Cardiology to treat stage 1 hypertension (systolic blood pressure [SBP] >130 or diastolic blood pressure [DBP] >80 mm Hg), maintain a higher degree of observation for women who have stage 1 hypertension, as there is some data to suggest higher risk of complications, including preeclampsia and eclampsia.

- There is no validated screening tool to predict the development of preeclampsia or eclampsia, therefore a high level of suspicion should be maintained for all pregnant patients presenting with new-onset hypertension or proteinuria.

- Early initiation of antihypertensive medication within 30 to 60 min, or as soon as reasonably possible, for women with severe range hypertension (SBP $\geq$160 mm Hg or DBP $\geq$110 mm Hg) can prevent serious fetal and maternal complications.

- All patients who present with preeclampsia with severe features or eclampsia should be treated with intravenous magnesium bolus and drip, and subsequently monitored for magnesium toxicity.

- Postpartum patients who present to the Emergency Department with new-onset hypertension, preeclampsia, or eclampsia should be assessed by an obstetrician.

DISCLOSURE

N. Coggins and S. Lai have no disclosures to share.

REFERENCES

1. Kassebaum B, Dandona H. Global, regional, and national levels of maternal mortality, 1990–2015: a systematic analysis for the Global Burden of Disease Study 2015. Lancet 2016;388(10053):1775–812. Available from: https://scholars. okstate.edu/en/publications/erratum-global-regional-and-national-levels-of-maternal-mortality.

2. Wagner SJ, Barac S, Garovic VD. Hypertensive pregnancy disorders: current concepts. J Clin Hypertens 2007;9(7):560–6.
3. Fingar K.R., Mabry-Hernandez I., Ngo-Metzger Q., et al., Delivery Hospitalizations Involving Preeclampsia and Eclampsia, 2005–2014. In: Healthcare Cost and Utilization Project (HCUP) Statistical Briefs [Internet]. Rockville (MD): Agency for Healthcare Research and Quality (US); 2006 Feb–. Statistical Brief #222. 2017.
4. Teng H, Wang Y, Han B, et al. Gestational systolic blood pressure trajectories and risk of adverse maternal and perinatal outcomes in Chinese women. BMC Pregnancy Childbirth 2021;21(1):155.
5. Bakker R, Steegers EAP, Hofman A, et al. Blood pressure in different gestational trimesters, fetal growth, and the risk of adverse birth outcomes: the generation R study. Am J Epidemiol 2011;174(7):797–806.
6. Hitti J, Sienas L, Walker S, et al. Contribution of hypertension to severe maternal morbidity. Am J Obstet Gynecol 2018;219(4):405.e1–7.
7. Whelton PK, Carey RM. The 2017 Clinical Practice Guideline for High Blood Pressure. JAMA 2017;318(21):2073–4.
8. Bateman BT, Bansil P, Hernandez-Diaz S, et al. Prevalence, trends, and outcomes of chronic hypertension: a nationwide sample of delivery admissions. Am J Obstet Gynecol 2012;206(2):134, e1–8.
9. Sibai BM, Lindheimer M, Hauth J, et al. Risk factors for preeclampsia, abruptio placentae, and adverse neonatal outcomes among women with chronic hypertension. National Institute of Child Health and Human Development Network of Maternal-Fetal Medicine Units. N Engl J Med 1998;339(10):667–71.
10. Buchbinder A, Sibai BM, Caritis S, et al. Adverse perinatal outcomes are significantly higher in severe gestational hypertension than in mild preeclampsia. Am J Obstet Gynecol 2002;186(1):66–71.
11. Ferrer RL, Sibai BM, Mulrow CD, et al. Management of mild chronic hypertension during pregnancy: a review. Obstet Gynecol 2000;96(5 Pt 2):849–60.
12. Vigil-De Gracia P, Lasso M, Montufar-Rueda C. Perinatal outcome in women with severe chronic hypertension during the second half of pregnancy. Int J Gynaecol Obstet 2004;85(2):139–44.
13. American College of Obstetricians and Gynecologists' Committee on Practice Bulletins—Obstetrics. ACOG Practice Bulletin No. 203: Chronic Hypertension in Pregnancy. Obstet Gynecol 2019;133(1):e26–50.
14. Croke L. Gestational Hypertension and Preeclampsia: A Practice Bulletin from ACOG. Am Fam Physician 2019;100(10):649–50.
15. Hypertension in pregnancy. Report of the American College of Obstetricians and Gynecologists' Task Force on Hypertension in Pregnancy. Obstet Gynecol 2013; 122(5):1122–31.
16. Kirshon B, Wasserstrum N, Cotton DB. Should continuous hydralazine infusions be utilized in severe pregnancy-induced hypertension? Am J Perinatol 1991; 8(3):206–8.
17. Begum MR, Quadir E, Begum A, et al. Management of hypertensive emergencies of pregnancy by hydralazine bolus injection vs continuous drip–a comparative study. Medscape Womens Health 2002;7(5):1.
18. Magee LA, Cham C, Waterman EJ, et al. Hydralazine for treatment of severe hypertension in pregnancy: meta-analysis. BMJ 2003;327(7421):955–60.
19. Sibai BM. Diagnosis and management of gestational hypertension and preeclampsia. Obstet Gynecol 2003;102(1):181–92.

20. Gestational Hypertension and Preeclampsia. ACOG Practice Bulletin Summary, Number 222. Obstet Gynecol 2020;135(6):1492–5.

21. Vermillion ST, Scardo JA, Newman RB, et al. A randomized, double-blind trial of oral nifedipine and intravenous labetalol in hypertensive emergencies of pregnancy. Am J Obstet Gynecol 1999;181(4):858–61.

22. Saudan P, Brown MA, Buddle ML, et al. Does gestational hypertension become pre-eclampsia? Br J Obstet Gynaecol 1998;105(11):1177–84.

23. Barton JR, O'brien JM, Bergauer NK, et al. Mild gestational hypertension remote from term: progression and outcome. Am J Obstet Gynecol 2001;184(5):979–83.

24. Magee LA, von Dadelszen P, Bohun CM, et al. Serious perinatal complications of non-proteinuric hypertension: an international, multicentre, retrospective cohort study. J Obstet Gynaecol Can 2003;25(5):372–82.

25. Lisonkova S, Joseph KS. Incidence of preeclampsia: risk factors and outcomes associated with early- versus late-onset disease. Am J Obstet Gynecol 2013; 209(6):544.e1–12.

26. Report of the National High Blood Pressure Education Program Working Group on High Blood Pressure in Pregnancy. Am J Obstet Gynecol 2000;183(1):S1–22.

27. Kuo VS, Koumantakis G, Gallery ED. Proteinuria and its assessment in normal and hypertensive pregnancy. Am J Obstet Gynecol 1992;167(3):723–8.

28. Morris RK, Riley RD, Doug M, et al. Diagnostic accuracy of spot urinary protein and albumin to creatinine ratios for detection of significant proteinuria or adverse pregnancy outcome in patients with suspected pre-eclampsia: systematic review and meta-analysis. BMJ 2012;345:e4342.

29. Thomson AM, Hytten FE, Billewicz WZ. The epidemiology of oedema during pregnancy. J Obstet Gynaecol Br Commonw 1967;74(1):1–10.

30. Cunningham FG, Gary Cunningham F, Gant NF, et al. Williams Obstetrics, 21st Edition [Internet]. J Midwifery Women's Health 2003;48(5):369.

31. Fox R, Kitt J, Leeson P, et al. Preeclampsia: Risk Factors, Diagnosis, Management, and the Cardiovascular Impact on the Offspring. J Clin Med Res [Internet] 2019;8:10.

32. Sibai BM. The HELLP syndrome (hemolysis, elevated liver enzymes, and low platelets): much ado about nothing? Am J Obstet Gynecol 1990;162(2):311–6.

33. Tomsen TR. HELLP syndrome (hemolysis, elevated liver enzymes, and low platelets) presenting as generalized malaise. Am J Obstet Gynecol 1995;172(6): 1876–8, discussion 1878–80.

34. Leeman L, Dresang LT, Fontaine P. Hypertensive Disorders of Pregnancy. Am Fam Physician 2016;93(2):121–7.

35. Sibai BM. Diagnosis, prevention, and management of eclampsia. Obstet Gynecol 2005;105(2):402–10.

36. Cooray SD, Edmonds SM, Tong S, et al. Characterization of symptoms immediately preceding eclampsia. Obstet Gynecol 2011;118(5):995–9.

37. Berhan Y, Berhan A. Should magnesium sulfate be administered to women with mild pre-eclampsia? A systematic review of published reports on eclampsia. J Obstet Gynaecol Res 2015;41(6):831–42.

38. Sibai BM, Stella CL. Diagnosis and management of atypical preeclampsia-eclampsia. Am J Obstet Gynecol 2009;200(5):481, e1–7.

39. Jaatinen N, Ekholm E. Eclampsia in Finland; 2006 to 2010. Acta Obstet Gynecol Scand 2016;95(7):787–92.

40. Vousden N, Lawley E, Seed PT, et al. Incidence of eclampsia and related complications across 10 low- and middle-resource geographical regions: Secondary analysis of a cluster randomised controlled trial. Plos Med 2019;16(3):e1002775.

41. Wagner SJ, Acquah LA, Lindell EP, et al. Posterior reversible encephalopathy syndrome and eclampsia: pressing the case for more aggressive blood pressure control. Mayo Clin Proc 2011;86(9):851–6.
42. Zeeman GG. Neurologic complications of pre-eclampsia. Semin Perinatol 2009; 33(3):166–72.
43. Sibai BM. Chronic hypertension in pregnancy. Obstet Gynecol 2002;100(2): 369–77.
44. Chappell LC, Enye S, Seed P, et al. Adverse perinatal outcomes and risk factors for preeclampsia in women with chronic hypertension: a prospective study. Hypertension 2008;51(4):1002–9.
45. Sutton EF, Hauspurg A, Caritis SN, et al. Maternal Outcomes Associated With Lower Range Stage 1 Hypertension. Obstet Gynecol 2018;132(4):843–9.
46. Cnossen JS, de Ruyter-Hanhijärvi H, van der Post JAM, et al. Accuracy of serum uric acid determination in predicting pre-eclampsia: a systematic review. Acta Obstet Gynecol Scand 2006;85(5):519–25.
47. Thangaratinam S, Ismail KMK, Sharp S, et al. Tests in Prediction of Pre-eclampsia Severity review group. Accuracy of serum uric acid in predicting complications of pre-eclampsia: a systematic review. BJOG 2006;113(4):369–78.
48. Livingston JR, Payne B, Brown M, et al. Uric Acid as a predictor of adverse maternal and perinatal outcomes in women hospitalized with preeclampsia. J Obstet Gynaecol Can 2014;36(10):870–7.
49. Roberge S, Nicolaides K, Demers S, et al. The role of aspirin dose on the prevention of preeclampsia and fetal growth restriction: systematic review and meta-analysis. Am J Obstet Gynecol 2017;216(2):110–20, e6.
50. Meher S, Duley L, Hunter K, et al. Antiplatelet therapy before or after 16 weeks' gestation for preventing preeclampsia: an individual participant data meta-analysis. Am J Obstet Gynecol 2017;216(2):121–8, e2.
51. Altman D, Carroli G, Duley L, et al. Do women with pre-eclampsia, and their babies, benefit from magnesium sulphate? The Magpie Trial: a randomised placebo-controlled trial. Lancet 2002;359(9321):1877–90.
52. Duley L, Henderson-Smart DJ, Walker GJ, et al. Magnesium sulphate versus diazepam for eclampsia. Cochrane Database Syst Rev 2010;12:CD000127.
53. Duley L, Gülmezoglu AM, Henderson-Smart DJ, et al. Magnesium sulphate and other anticonvulsants for women with pre-eclampsia. Cochrane Database Syst Rev 2010;11:CD000025.
54. Cahill AG, Macones GA, Odibo AO, et al. Magnesium for seizure prophylaxis in patients with mild preeclampsia. Obstet Gynecol 2007;110(3):601–7.
55. Webster LM, Conti-Ramsden F, Seed PT, et al. Impact of Antihypertensive Treatment on Maternal and Perinatal Outcomes in Pregnancy Complicated by Chronic Hypertension: A Systematic Review and Meta-Analysis. J Am Heart Assoc [Internet] 2017;6(5):e005526.
56. Magee LA, von Dadelszen P, Singer J, et al. The CHIPS Randomized Controlled Trial (Control of Hypertension in Pregnancy Study): Is Severe Hypertension Just an Elevated Blood Pressure? Hypertension 2016;68(5):1153–9.
57. Abalos E, Duley L, Steyn DW, et al. Antihypertensive drug therapy for mild to moderate hypertension during pregnancy. Cochrane Database Syst Rev 2018; 10:CD002252.
58. Tita AT, Szychowski JM, Boggess K, et al. Treatment for Mild Chronic Hypertension during Pregnancy. N Engl J Med 2022;386(19):1781–92.
59. ElFarra J, Bean C, Martin JN Jr. Management of Hypertensive Crisis for the Obstetrician/Gynecologist. Obstet Gynecol Clin North Am 2016;43(4):623–37.

60. Magee LA. Treating hypertension in women of child-bearing age and during pregnancy. Drug Saf 2001;24(6):457–74.

61. Seely EW, Ecker J. Clinical practice. Chronic hypertension in pregnancy. N Engl J Med 2011;365(5):439–46.

62. Xie R-H, Guo Y, Krewski D, et al. Beta-blockers increase the risk of being born small for gestational age or of being institutionalised during infancy. BJOG 2014;121(9):1090–6.

63. Cockburn J, Moar VA, Ounsted M, et al. Final report of study on hypertension during pregnancy: the effects of specific treatment on the growth and development of the children. Lancet 1982;1(8273):647–9.

Emergency Delivery

Michele Callahan, MD

KEYWORDS

- Precipitous labor • Emergency department • Emergency delivery
- Shoulder dystocia • Breech delivery

KEY POINTS

- Every ED should have supplies readily available for a possible imminent vaginal delivery, including supplies necessary to resuscitate 2 potential patients—mother and neonate.
- Knowledge of maneuvers used to manage complicated deliveries (such as shoulder dystocia, breech presentation, and cord prolapse) is a critical skill set for emergency physicians.
- Immediately upon recognizing a shoulder dystocia, the entire team should be notified out loud, and McRoberts maneuver (with suprapubic pressure) should be initiated.
- Breech deliveries should be handled in a "hands off" manner as much as possible to prevent worsening head entrapment and fetal asphyxiation.
- Every patient delivering in the ED should have active management of labor, which includes routine administration of uterotonic medication(s) such as oxytocin, in order to minimize blood loss and prevent the morbidity and mortality associated with postpartum hemorrhage.

BACKGROUND

Managing a precipitous delivery in the emergency department (ED) is a stress-inducing scenario for most emergency physicians. Although most women presenting to the ED in labor will be appropriate for transfer to the labor and delivery unit, there is a subset of patients that will deliver imminently, and who will therefore require delivery and stabilization in the ED. Similarly, although most infants will be born without difficulty and will require no resuscitative efforts, a small subset of infants will require further resuscitation. The incidence of ED deliveries is not well reported in the literature. The most recent birth data from 2021 shows that approximately 10% of births were preterm (<37 weeks gestation).[1]

Precipitous labor is defined as labor that lasts less than 3 hours from the onset of regular contractions to delivery of the infant. In 2015, the Centers for Disease Control and Prevention reported a precipitous delivery incidence of approximately 3% in the United States.[2] The incidence of ED deliveries is unknown and not well reported.

Department of Emergency Medicine, University of Maryland School of Medicine, 110 South Paca Street, 6th Floor, Suite 200, Baltimore, MD 21201, USA
E-mail address: mcallahan@som.umaryland.edu

Emerg Med Clin N Am 41 (2023) 281–294
https://doi.org/10.1016/j.emc.2022.12.002
0733-8627/23/© 2022 Elsevier Inc. All rights reserved.

INTRODUCTION

This article will review vaginal delivery and neonatal resuscitation within the ED and will include discussion of possible complications (such as breech delivery, shoulder dystocia, and postpartum hemorrhage [PPH]) and how to adeptly manage these clinical scenarios.

It is necessary to anticipate the need to manage and resuscitate 2 patients, both the mother and the infant. Although most infants will be healthy and born without complication, a very small subset of neonates may require resuscitation such as chest compressions and supplemental oxygen administration. Past data estimates that 10% of neonates will require some additional level of breathing assistance at the time of birth, with 1% requiring intensive cardiopulmonary resuscitation.[3]

Emergency physicians should feel comfortable managing an uncomplicated delivery and should also be aware of maneuvers necessary for managing more complicated birth scenarios such as shoulder dystocia, nuchal cord, and breech positioning.

The Emergency Medical Treatment and Labor Act requires a medical screening examination and stabilization of medical emergencies before transfer. A woman in labor is considered to be unstable if there are signs of impending labor (ie, if there is not enough time to transfer her to another facility before delivery occurs). It is prudent for the emergency physician to quickly determine whether a patient's labor is imminent, or whether rapid transfer to the nearest hospital with obstetric care is possible.

GENERAL APPROACH TO EMERGENCY DEPARTMENT DELIVERY

All patients who present to the ED with signs of labor should undergo a thorough but rapid evaluation that includes obtaining IV access, maternal vital signs, measurement of fetal heart tones, and a sterile vaginal examination to determine if there is any crowning or cervical dilation. If there is significant vaginal bleeding, and no obvious evidence of crowning, attempts should be made to obtain an ultrasound that will evaluate specifically for placenta previa. Any additional manipulation (such as a speculum examination) could cause significant hemorrhage in a patient with placenta previa.

Signs of imminent labor include intense contractions that are regularly and closely spaced, a patient feeling the need to push or bear down, and crowning (fetal head/presenting part visible at the introitus). If these signs exist, the provider should prepare for delivery in the ED because the patient is too far along to be transferred elsewhere.

Necessary history to elicit from the patient includes gravidity and parity, dating of the current pregnancy, the presence or absence of prenatal care, the number of babies expected to be delivered (ie, twins), any complications thus far in the pregnancy, and any pertinent maternal medical problems. Complications of the current pregnancy would include knowledge of any abnormal placentation (such as placenta previa), uncontrolled hypertension or preeclampsia, and gestational diabetes.

If the dating of the pregnancy is unknown, a due date can be calculated based on the first day of the last menstrual period. Using this date, subtracting 3 months, and adding 1 week will provide an estimated due date. The estimated gestation can also be determined using the gravid uterus-at approximately 20 weeks gestation, the uterus is palpable at the level of the umbilicus. The uterus rises 1 to 2 cm every additional week of gestation.

It is then helpful to obtain a history of the onset of labor symptoms—the onset and frequency of contractions, whether there has been any vaginal bleeding or leakage of fluid to indicate ruptured membranes, and whether there continues to be fetal movement appreciated by the mother.

Ultrasound is a useful adjunct when evaluating a patient in precipitous labor within the ED. It will allow the emergency physician to obtain dating of the pregnancy (based on a variety of measurements such as biparietal diameter, femur length, or abdominal circumference), to determine if there are multiple gestations, and to obtain a fetal heart rate. The ultrasound is also useful in visualizing the presenting part—the majority of deliveries will involve a cephalic (head down) presentation, but in some cases the positioning will indicate a breech delivery is imminent.

A sterile speculum examination should be performed to determine if there is evidence of rupture of membranes (ROM), to assess for cervical dilation and effacement (thinning), and to evaluate for the presenting fetal part. In 95% of vaginal deliveries, the baby will present cephalic (head down).[4]

As mentioned above, with obvious significant bleeding, an ultrasound should be attempted to evaluate for placenta previa before the speculum examination. Signs of ruptured membranes include pooling of liquid in the vaginal vault, a positive nitrazine test (a specimen of vaginal fluid with a pH greater than 6 is likely amniotic, indicated ROM), and ferning of fluid on a microscope slide. It is helpful to obtain history about when the patient thought their membranes ruptured—that is, when their water broke—as this can point toward any increased risk of infection.

EMERGENCY DELIVERY SUPPLIES

Most EDs will have previously prepared delivery kits that should include all supplies necessary for a precipitous delivery. It is important for the emergency physician to be aware of the resources available to them, both with regards to supplies as well as available consultants. It is particularly important to have an early involvement of obstetrics (or general surgery if your facility does not have an obstetrician), neonatologists, and other support staff.

A basic list of supplies that will be needed for the delivery itself (**Box 1**) includes sterile gloves, a scalpel, surgical scissors, hemostats, cord clamps, towels, and absorbable sutures. Supplies for neonatal resuscitation (**Box 2**) should also be prepared in a nearby kit and ideally stored on or near an infant warmer/isolette.

MANAGING AN UNCOMPLICATED DELIVERY

If a delivery is imminent, a delivery kit (and neonatal resuscitation supplies) should be nearby and readily available. Sterile gloves should be donned and towels used to drape the perineum. If time allows, povidone-iodine can be used to cleanse the

Box 1
Emergency delivery kit
Sterile gloves
Gauze sponges
Scalpel
Surgical scissors
Hemostats
Umbilical cord clamps
Towels
Absorbable sutures

Box 2
Neonatal resuscitation supplies

Infant isolette/warmer

Blankets and/or towels, hat

Occlusive wrap (polyethylene)

Infant face mask

Bulb suction, suction catheter, and tubing

Bag valve mask, LMA size 1

Endotracheal tubes (+stylet) in multiple sizes-2.5 to 4

Laryngoscopes- Miller 00, 0, and 1

Portable oxygen source

O_2 saturation probe, ECG leads

Supplies for IV/IO/umbilical vein access

Pediatric code cart

---

perineum and vagina. As the fetal head emerges from the introitus, the emergency physician should place a gloved hand at the perineum and provide gentle upward pressure on the fetal chin as well as gentle counterpressure on the occiput to guide delivery of the fetal head and minimize perineal trauma. Although routine suctioning of the infant's mouth and nose continues to be common practice at this juncture of the delivery, it is no longer routinely recommended by pediatric guidelines.[5]

Once the head has been delivered, the physician should evaluate for whether a nuchal cord (umbilical cord around the fetal neck) is present and slip it over the infant's head if so. If unable to be loosened or passed over the head, the cord can be clamped on 2 sides and then the physician can carefully cut between the 2 clamps.

After delivery of the head, the fetal body will rotate to face the maternal thigh. At this time, gentle downward traction helps to guide delivery of the anterior shoulder, followed by gentle upward traction to deliver the posterior shoulder. Care should be taken to hold on tightly to the infant as the body is delivered. The infant should then be warmed, dried, and stimulated, at which time the need for further resuscitation is assessed.

The newest neonatal resuscitation guidelines recommend delayed cord clamping after birth for at least 30 to 60 seconds in all infants not requiring further resuscitation. Benefits have been seen for preterm births (decreased need for blood transfusion and lower incidence of necrotizing enterocolitis and intraventricular hemorrhage) as well as term births (increased hemoglobin levels and iron stores in early life).[6] If there is a disruption to the placental circulation (such as concern for abruption), the cord should be clamped immediately.

If the delivery is uncomplicated and no neonatal resuscitation is required, it is appropriate (and beneficial) to offer immediate skin-to-skin by placing the infant on the mother's chest. Skin-to-skin contact has numerous benefits, including regulation of the infant glucose levels, breathing, and heart rate. It also stimulates oxytocin release in both the infant and mother, encouraging bonding while also allowing uterine contraction and minimizing postpartum bleeding. Early encouragement of breastfeeding is supported by the World Health Organization (WHO), and efforts should be made to offer this option to the mother as soon as possible.[7]

Delivery of the Placenta

The American College of Obstetricians and Gynecologists (ACOG) and the WHO have targeted active management of the third stage of labor as a critical intervention in preventing PPH. Active management includes a combination of routine uterotonic administration (typically, oxytocin), controlled cord traction, and uterine massage.[8]

After the umbilical cord has been clamped and cut, gentle traction can be applied to guide detachment of the placenta. Signs of placental separation from the uterus include a gush of blood, lengthening of the umbilical cord, and the uterus contracting and rising within the abdomen. While providing traction to the cord, the physician should also apply gentle counterpressure to the uterus with uterine massage. There should be no forceful pulling because the placenta can tear and cause significant persistent bleeding if retained tissue is present.

A variety of uterotonic medications are available, with the most commonly used (and readily available) being oxytocin. Prophylactic oxytocin in a dose of 10 mg IV (diluted, given as an infusion) or 10 mg IM should be part of every ED delivery. The timing of initiation of oxytocin has not yet been adequately studied but it should be given routinely= at the time of placental delivery, if not already given earlier.

COMPLICATED DELIVERY MANEUVERS
Maneuvers: Shoulder Dystocia

ACOG defines shoulder dystocia as an obstetric emergency when there is failure to deliver the fetal shoulder(s) with gentle downward traction on the fetal head. This requires rapid identification and additional maneuvers to facilitate delivery. The incidence of shoulder dystocia among vaginal deliveries ranges from 0.2% to 3%.[9] Risk factors such as gestational diabetes, obesity, or a prior delivery complicated by shoulder dystocia, have a poor negative predictive value for whether a dystocia will be present. Risk factors can only predict a shoulder dystocia in 50% to 70% of cases.[10] As shoulder dystocia is an unpredictable occurrence, emergency physicians must be adept at both diagnosing a dystocia and understanding which maneuvers to use when attempting delivery.

Emergency physicians should suspect a shoulder dystocia if the fetal head retracts against the maternal perineum (known as the "turtle sign") during delivery.

The first step when recognizing that a shoulder dystocia is present is to call for additional help. This should include (but is not limited to) additional nursing staff, secondary emergency physicians (if multiple are on shift simultaneously), obstetricians and/or general surgeons, and the neonatal resuscitation team. The concern for shoulder dystocia should be clearly voiced, and a timer should be started in order to track the time for head delivery to occur. The patient should be instructed not to push because this will worsen impaction.

The most commonly effective maneuver, and the one to perform first, is the McRoberts maneuver (**Fig. 1**). This involves hyperflexion and abduction of the maternal hips. Staff members can assist in positioning by each holding one of the mother's legs, and/ or applying gentle and consistent suprapubic -not fundal- pressure. It is important to avoid fundal pressure because this can worsen fetal impaction at the pubic symphysis. A combination of McRoberts maneuver and suprapubic pressure has been found to relieve approximately two-third of shoulder dystocias.[11] If there is no relief with McRoberts and suprapubic pressure, delivery of the posterior arm can be attempted (**Fig. 2**). To deliver the posterior arm, the physician places one hand into the vagina and flexes the posterior fetal arm at the elbow, until the forearm or hand can be used to sweep the arm across the fetal chest. This will allow the posterior arm and shoulder to be delivered.

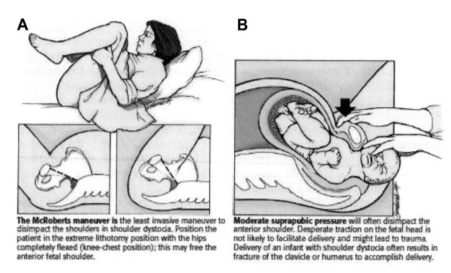

A

B

The McRoberts maneuver is the least invasive maneuver to disimpact the shoulders in shoulder dystocia. Position the patient in the extreme lithotomy position with the hips completely flexed (knee-chest position); this may free the anterior fetal shoulder.

Moderate suprapubic pressure will often disimpact the anterior shoulder. Desperate traction on the fetal head is not likely to facilitate delivery and might lead to trauma. Delivery of an infant with shoulder dystocia often results in fracture of the clavicle or humerus to accomplish delivery.

Fig. 1. The McRoberts maneuver involves hyperflexion at the hips and knee-to-chest positioning (A). It may also include suprapubic pressure (B), which can disimpact the shoulder from underneath the pubic symphysis. (From: Susan M. Lanni, Robert Gherman, Bernard Gonik, Chapter 17 - Malpresentations, Editor(s): Steven G. Gabbe, Jennifer R. Niebyl, Joe Leigh Simpson, Mark B. Landon, Henry L. Galan, Eric R.M. Jauniaux, Deborah A. Driscoll, Vincenzo Berghella, William A. Grobman, Obstetrics: Normal and Problem Pregnancies (Seventh Edition), Elsevier, 2017, Pages 368-394.)

There are also several rotational maneuvers to attempt, including the Woods' Screw maneuver and the Rubin maneuver. The Woods' Screw maneuver (**Fig. 3**) involves inserting 2 fingers into the posterior aspect of the vagina and applying pressure to the anterior surface of the posterior shoulder to rotate the infant 180°. The Rubin technique is similar but involves pressure placed on the posterior surface of the posterior shoulder in an attempt to adduct the shoulder.[12]

The patient can also be transitioned to an all-fours position (the Gaskin maneuver) on her hands and knees with attempts made to apply downward traction on the posterior shoulder or upward traction on the anterior shoulder. Attempting the above maneuvers should lead to delivery in 99% of cases.[11]

Additional, and less ideal, management options include performing an episiotomy and the Zavanelli maneuver -pushing the fetal head inward and proceeding with cesarean section-which is only an option if a surgeon is available to perform this.

Common sequelae of shoulder dystocia (and subsequent difficult delivery) include increased incidences of PPH, fourth-degree lacerations, anal sphincter injuries, and additional injuries such as to the urethra and bladder. Neonatal complications most commonly include brachial plexus injuries (often with a subsequent Erb or Klumpke Palsy), fractures of the humerus and clavicle, and of course the more feared complications of hypoxic-ischemic encephalopathy or death.[12]

Maneuvers: Breech Position

Breech presentation refers to a delivery in which the feet or buttocks are the presenting part; this is the most common type of malpresentation. There are several variations of breech positioning (frank breech, complete breech, incomplete breech, and footling breech) based on relative position of the hips, knees, feet, and buttocks.

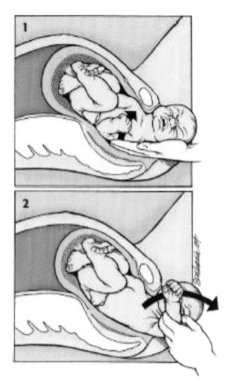

D
Posterior shoulder delivery. Insert a hand and sweep the posterior arm across the chest and over the perineum. Take care to distribute the pressure evenly across the humerus to avoid unnecessary fracture.

Fig. 2. Delivery of the posterior arm/shoulder by sweeping the arm across the infant's chest can change the diameter of the presenting part and allow for relief of fetal impaction in the event of a shoulder dystocia. (*From*: Susan M. Lanni, Robert Gherman, Bernard Gonik, Chapter 17 - Malpresentations, Editor(s): Steven G. Gabbe, Jennifer R. Niebyl, Joe Leigh Simpson, Mark B. Landon, Henry L. Galan, Eric R.M. Jauniaux, Deborah A. Driscoll, Vincenzo Berghella, William A. Grobman, Obstetrics: Normal and Problem Pregnancies (Seventh Edition), Elsevier, 2017, Pages 368-394.)

Approximately 3% to 4% of deliveries are breech. Breech presentation is associated with higher morbidity and mortality for both mother and fetus.[13] For patients with prenatal care, breech positioning is an indication for cesarean delivery. In a precipitous ED delivery, particularly in ED settings where the option for surgical intervention is not readily available, there are several maneuvers that can be attempted to facilitate a vaginal breech delivery.

In general, breech deliveries should be more "hands off" than a typical cephalic delivery, to allow the fetal presenting part to maximally dilate the cervix.[14] **Figs. 4** and **5** outlines the steps associated with vaginal breech delivery, if cesarean section is not an option. Fetal manipulation should generally be avoided until the fetus has spontaneously delivered to the level of the umbilicus—any tension on the infant can lead to head entrapment.[15] Once the fetus is visible to the level of the umbilicus, gently deliver the legs with the Pinard maneuver (flexing the knee by pressure applied to the inner

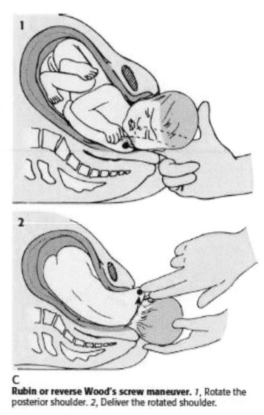

C
Rubin or reverse Wood's screw maneuver. *1,* Rotate the posterior shoulder. *2,* Deliver the rotated shoulder.

Fig. 3. Rotational maneuvers of the posterior and/or anterior shoulder can help to relieve fetal impaction in the event of a shoulder dystocia. (*From:* Lew GH, Pulia MS. Emergency Childbirth. Roberts and Hedges' Clinical Procedures in Emergency Medicine, 6e. Philadelphia, PA: Elsevier; 2014:1155-1179. Images used with permission.)

aspect of the knee, and then sweeping the leg out of the vagina). This can be repeated with the contralateral leg. Maintain gentle pressure and hold baby around the hips, making sure to avoid significant pressure on the abdomen because this can cause damage to abdominal organs. The sacrum should not be rotated into the anterior position, if not already in that orientation. Once the baby has delivered to the level of the scapula, the baby can be rotated sideways to allow for delivery of one arm, then rotated 180° to deliver the other arm. Next, rotation should occur to return the baby to sacrum anterior positioning. At this point, the Mauriceau maneuver can be performed to guide delivery of the fetal head. In this maneuver, the physician maneuvers one hand into the vagina and places gentle pressure to the fetal maxilla. This will allow for slight flexion of the fetal neck. At the same time, the physician's other hand is placed on the occiput for counterpressure, to avoid any abnormal traction on the fetal neck. While maintaining flexion at the neck, the physician can pull gently to deliver the fetal head.[16] It can be helpful to have a second person assist by putting gentle pressure on the pubic bone to assist with fetal head flexion.

Bedside ultrasound can be immensely helpful in visualizing the presenting part and making the diagnosis of an impending breech delivery, if the presenting part is not already externally visible.

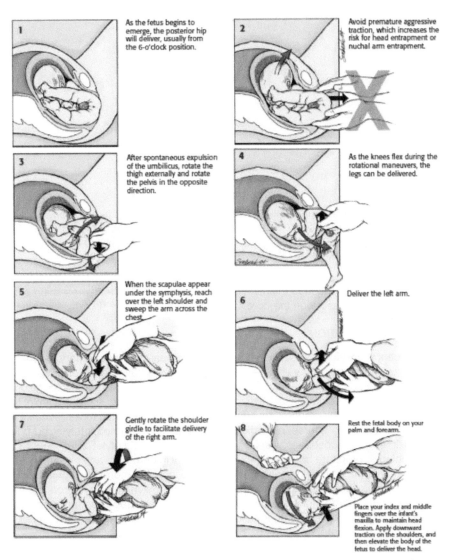

Fig. 4. Breech delivery involves a more hands-off approach, with maneuvers to gently assist the removal of the arms and legs. (*From*: Susan M. Lanni, Robert Gherman, Bernard Gonik, Chapter 17 - Malpresentations, Editor(s): Steven G. Gabbe, Jennifer R. Niebyl, Joe Leigh Simpson, Mark B. Landon, Henry L. Galan, Eric R.M. Jauniaux, Deborah A. Driscoll, Vincenzo Berghella, William A. Grobman, Obstetrics: Normal and Problem Pregnancies (Seventh Edition), Elsevier, 2017, Pages 368-394.)

Maneuvers: Umbilical Cord Prolapse

Umbilical cord prolapse is an obstetric emergency. In the ED, this may be visible as a loop of umbilical cord at the vaginal introitus or seen during a sterile speculum examination. The presence of a prolapse can threaten fetal oxygenation, leading to hypoxia and poor outcomes. If an umbilical cord prolapse is recognized, the patient should immediately be placed in a knee-to-chest position, and obstetric consultants should be contacted for a possible stat cesarean delivery. If the patient requires transport,

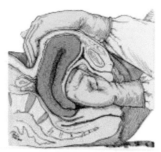

Use uterine massage to control postpartum bleeding.
Insert one hand into the vagina to compress the anterior uterine wall
while massaging the posterior aspect of the uterus through the
abdominal wall with the other hand.

Fig. 5. Patients with concern for PPH, particularly in the setting of uterine atony, should receive uterine massage in addition to uterotonic medications. (*From*: Lew GH, Pulia MS. Emergency Childbirth. Roberts and Hedges' Clinical Procedures in Emergency Medicine, 6e. Philadelphia, PA: Elsevier; 2014:1155-1179. Images used with permission.)

every effort should be made to maintain upward pressure on the fetal presenting part in order to relieve pressure on the cord.[17]

NEONATAL RESUSCITATION

The emergency physician should prepare for a neonatal resuscitation and have all necessary supplies readily available—many hospitals will have an isolette with kits for both delivery and neonatal resuscitation all together. Essential supplies for resuscitation of a neonate include an infant warmer, a kelly clamp and scissors, a blanket to dry/stimulate, bulb suction and/or suction catheters to be connected to wall suction, a supplementary oxygen source, a cardiorespiratory monitor, appropriately sized bag valve mask, and laryngoscopes with endotracheal tubes and a stylet.

Maintaining appropriate body temperature is critical in both term and preterm newborns. Hypothermia has been consistently shown to increase morbidity and mortality in preterm infants. Warming with blankets or using skin-to-skin may be appropriate for term infants but other techniques may be required for infants requiring further resuscitation. Additional warming methods include the use of plastic wrap (being sure to avoid the head/face), radiant warmers, and infant caps.

The newest guidelines recommend suctioning of the newborn only if the airway is obstructed or positive pressure ventilation is required. If meconium-stained amniotic fluid is present, intubation and endotracheal suctioning are only required in infants who need it for ventilation or airway obstruction (not all-comers).[5]

Infant heart rate should be monitored using a 3-lead electrocardiogram (ECG) in order to ensure accurate and continuous readings. Resuscitation should always begin with room air (21%) in infants requiring ventilation/oxygenation, only adding supplemental oxygen as needed to obtain appropriate saturations on pulse oximetry. If the infant's heart rate is less than 60 bmp after a 30-second trial of positive-pressure ventilation, chest compressions should be initiated. Intubation of the infant should be considered at this time.[5]

A more detailed discussion of neonatal resuscitation can be found by reviewing the neonatal resuscitation program guidelines, which are updated regularly. A review of calculating APGAR scores (which stands for Appearance, Pulse, Grimace, Activity, and Respiration), routinely done at 0 and 5 minutes, can be found in **Table 1**. APGAR

Table 1
APGAR scoring system

Score	Appearance	Pulse	Grimace	Activity	Respirations
0	Cyanotic/pale	Absent	No response	Flaccid	Absent
1	Peripheral cyanosis	<100 bpm	Minimal response	Some flexion	Slow, irregular
2	Pink	>100 bpm	Active response (sneeze, cry, cough)	Active movement	Vigorous cry

scoring is a standardized method for assessing an infant's adaptation to extrauterine life, and their response to resuscitation (if needed). If the APGAR score remains less than 7 at the 5-minute mark, scoring should be continued every 5 minutes for 20 minutes.

POSTPARTUM HEMORRHAGE

As mentioned previously, it is recommended to empirically treat with oxytocin during the third stage of labor in order to minimize blood loss. With any delivery, physicians should be prepared to intervene if there is any concern of PPH.

In 2021, the American College of Obstetricians and Gynecologists updated their definition of PPH: cumulative blood loss of more than 1000 mL or blood loss that is accompanied by signs and symptoms of hypovolemia within 24 hours. The most common cause for PPH is uterine atony but other causes such as cervical laceration, retained products of conception, and abnormal placentation can be seen as well. The emergency physician should have a high level of suspicion for PPH in order to initiate treatment early- signs of significant blood loss such as tachycardia and hypotension can be delayed in an otherwise young and healthy individual. If there is any concern for PPH, treatment should be immediately initiated.

A helpful mnemonic when thinking about causes of heavy postpartum bleeding is the "4 Ts"—tone, trauma, tissue, and thrombin. **Table 2** outlines the common causes and treatment strategies. The most common cause for PPH is uterine atony (abnormal tone).[8] When suspecting uterine atony, a combination of uterine massage, bimanual compression, and uterotonic drugs should be used. Alternate causes for significant bleeding include trauma (such as cervical lacerations or uterine rupture), retained placental tissue, and abnormalities of coagulation. Each of these causes requires a slightly different management in the ED, such as manual removal of retained tissue or replacement of clotting factors through transfusion. It is important to have surgical specialists involved in management at this point because the patient may require surgical intervention if the bleeding continues to be uncontrolled.

Table 2
Postpartum hemorrhage

Cause	Etiologies	Management
Tone	Uterine atony	Uterotonic medications, bimanual massage
Trauma	Lacerations, uterine rupture, uterine inversion	Packing, surgical repair
Tissue	Retained tissue, abnormal placentation	Manual removal, curettage/surgical management
Thrombin	Coagulopathy	Transfusion of blood products, clotting factors

Additional uterotonic medications beyond oxytocin include methylergonovine, PGE1 (Prostaglandin E1, or misoprostol), and 15-methyl prostaglandin $F_{2\alpha}$ (Hemabate). These medications can be used in combination if needed to control bleeding.

Vaginal and perineal lacerations may lead to excessive bleeding. The emergency physician should evaluate for any obvious lacerations or tears and attempt to pack these areas to control bleeding, or if no surgical colleagues are readily available, the emergency physician can attempt a temporary repair with absorbable sutures such as chromic gut.

Some causes of PPH will only be definitely managed in the operating room; therefore, it is important to have surgical consultants involved early on. For example, retained placental tissue can often be removed manually at the bedside. However, there are instances of abnormal placentation, such as placenta accreta, where more invasive procedures such as hysteroscopy or curettage are necessary. In severe cases of PPH, hysterectomy may be required as a life-saving procedure when more conservative measures have failed. The involvement of interventional radiology for uterine artery embolization may also be useful in cases of uncontrolled bleeding.

Management of PPH should also include resuscitation with blood products as necessary, ideally O Rh-negative blood. With significant blood loss, it is possible for patients to develop disseminated intravascular coagulation (DIC), a life-threatening consumptive coagulopathy.

Massive transfusion is defined as transfusion of more than 10 units of packed red blood cells in 24 hours, transfusion of more than 4 units within 1 hour with ongoing need for additional blood anticipated, or replacing a complete blood volume.[8] When initiating a massive transfusion protocol, the recommended initial ratio is 1:1:1 (pRBC: fresh frozen plasma: platelets). If the patient is found to be in DIC, the emergency physician should consider administering cryoprecipitate as well.

Tranexamic acid is an antifibrinolytic agent with proposed utility in patients with PPH. The WOMAN trial[18,19] reported a reduction in mortality rates from obstetric hemorrhage when given within 3 hours of birth. The data still remain limited but emergency physicians can consider a dose of 10,000 mg IV if bleeding is uncontrolled.

As PPH complicates 4% to 6% of all deliveries and causes a significant increase in maternal morbidity and mortality, it is important for emergency physicians to recognize PPH and be aware of the different management strategies available to them.[11]

SUMMARY

Although most pregnant women presenting to the ED in labor will be suitable for transfer to the obstetric unit, a subset of these patients will require imminent management and delivery in the ED. The ED team should have protocols in place, with appropriate supplies available, to manage a delivery and potential resuscitation of both mother and infant. Although most deliveries will be uncomplicated and the infant will not require anything beyond routine postnatal care, complications do occur and the emergency physician should be confident managing these scenarios.

CLINICS CARE POINTS

- Most patients presenting to the ED with an imminent delivery will require minimal significant intervention during and after delivery; a small subset of patients (both mother and infant) will require additional resuscitation beyond routine care. Approximately 10% of infants require additional breathing assistance, with 1% requiring more in-depth resuscitation.

- Recognition of shoulder dystocia should prompt the emergency physician to immediately notify the team of their concern, quickly followed by initiation of the McRoberts maneuver with suprapubic pressure. If this fails to reduce the dystocia, additional maneuvers -rotational maneuvers, delivery of the posterior arm, and so forth- should then be attempted in rapid succession.

- Management of a breech delivery should involve a "hands off" approach until the infant has delivered spontaneously to the level of the umbilicus—this allows the presenting part to maximally dilate the cervix and minimizes the risk of head entrapment. After this time, using the Pinard and Mauriceau maneuvers can help to guide delivery.

- It is imperative to actively manage the third stage of labor (delivery of the placenta) with a combination of uterotonic medications (most often oxytocin), uterine massage, and gentle cord traction. Routine use of uterotonic medications has been proven to minimize the risk of PPH and subsequent morbidity and mortality.

- When evaluating for possible causes of PPH, remember the 4 Ts: tone, trauma, tissue, and thrombin. Uterine atony is the most common cause and can be alleviated with a combination of uterotonic medications and bimanual uterine massage.

- Neonatal resuscitation guidelines are regularly updated and should be reviewed by emergency physicians regularly. The most updated guidelines no longer recommend routine suction of the infant at the time of birth, and recommend heart rate monitoring be done using a 3-lead ECG, in order to accurately guide resuscitative efforts.

DISCLOSURE

The author has no disclosures to make and no financial conflicts of interest.

REFERENCES

1. Hamilton BE, Martin JA, Osterman MJK. Births: Provisional Data for 2021. Vital Statistics Rapid Release. 2022. Available at. https://www.cdc.gov/nchs/data/vsrr/vsrr020.pdf.
2. Martin JA, Hamilton BE, Osterman MJ, et al. Births: Final data for 2013. Natl Vital Stat Rep 2015;64:1–65.
3. Aziz K, Lee HC, Escobedo MB, et al. Part 5: neonatal resuscitation: 2020 american heart association guidelines for cardiopulmonary resuscitation and emergency cardiovascular care. Circulation 2020;142(16_suppl_2):S524–50.
4. Kilpatrick S, Garrison E. Normal labor and delivery. In: Gabbe EG, Niebyl JR, Simpson JL, et al, editors. Obstetrics: normal and problem pregnancies. 7th edition. Philadelphia: Elsevier; 2017. p. 368–94.
5. Escobedo MB, Shah BA, Song C, et al. Recent recommendations and emerging science in neonatal resuscitation. Pediatr Clin North Am 2019;66(2):309–20.
6. Delayed umbilical cord clamping after birth. ACOG Committee Opinion No. 814. American College of Obstetricians and Gynecologists. Obstet Gynecol 2020;136:e100–6.
7. Crenshaw JT. Healthy Birth Practice #6: Keep Mother and Baby Together- It's Best for Mother, Baby, and Breastfeeding. J Perinat Educ 2014;23(4):211–7.
8. Committee on Practice Bulletins-Obstetrics. Practice Bulletin No. 183: Postpartum Hemorrhage. Obstet Gynecol 2017;130:e168.
9. Practice Bulletin No 178: Shoulder Dystocia. Obstet Gynecol 2017;129(5):e123–33.
10. Bothou A, Apostolidi DM, Tsikouras P, et al. Overview of techniques to manage shoulder dystocia during vaginal birth. Eur J Midwifery 2021;5:48.

11. Dahlke JD, Bhalwal A, Chauhan SP. Obstetric Emergencies: Shoulder Dystocia and Postpartum Hemorrhage. Obstet Gynecol Clin North Am 2017;44(2):231–43.
12. Del Portal DA, Horn AE, Vilke GM, et al. Emergency department management of shoulder dystocia. J Emerg Med 2014;46(3):378–82.
13. Pilliod RA, Caughey AB. Fetal malpresentation and malposition: diagnosis and management. Obstet Gynecol Clin North Am 2017;44(4):631–43.
14. Silver DW, Sabatino F. Precipitous and difficult deliveries. Emerg Med Clin North Am 2012;30(4):961–75.
15. Borhart J, Voss K. Precipitous labor and emergency department delivery. Emerg Med Clin North Am 2019;37(2):265–76.
16. Mercado J, Brea I, Mendez B, et al. Critical obstetric and gynecologic procedures in the emergency department. Emerg Med Clin North Am 2013;31(1):207–36.
17. Dooley-Hash S, Knoop KJ. Umbilical cord prolapse in emergency delivery. In: *The Atlas of Emergency Medicine*, 5. New York: McGraw Hill; 2021.
18. WOMAN Trial Collaborators. Effect of early tranexamic acid administration on mortality, hysterectomy, and other morbidities in women with post-partum haemorrhage (WOMAN): an international, randomised, double-blind, placebo-controlled trial. Lancet 2017;389(10084):2105–16, published correction appears in Lancet. 2017;389(10084):2104.
19. Lew GH, Pulia MS. Chapter 56:Emergency Childbirth. In: Roberts JR, Hedges JR, Custalow CB, et al, editors. Clinical Procedures in Emergency Medicine. edition 6. Philadelphia: Saunders; 2013. p. 1155–82.

Spontaneous and Complicated Therapeutic Abortion in the Emergency Department

Sara Manning, MD*, Diane Kuhn, MD, PhD

KEYWORDS

- Abortion • Early pregnancy loss • Septic abortion • Hemorrhage

KEY POINTS

- Spontaneous abortion affects nearly 1 in 5 recognized pregnancies, far above the perceived rate estimated by the lay public.
- Spontaneous abortion may be safely and effectively managed with expectant, medical, or surgical approaches.
- Complications of therapeutic abortion are rare and include incomplete or failed abortion, hemorrhage, septic abortion, and uterine perforation.
- The legal status of abortion in the United States is now determined at the state level introducing stark differences in abortion access across the country.

INTRODUCTION

Every year, more than a million patients seek pregnancy-related care in US emergency departments (EDs). These visits make pregnancy-related issues among the 10 most common reasons for seeking emergency care for reproductive-aged women.[1] Pregnancy-related visits include spontaneous and therapeutic abortion and their associated complications. Whether it is planned or unplanned, the end of a pregnancy is often a stressful and emotionally charged time for patients. Evidence regarding the ED patient experience with early pregnancy loss is limited but suggests an overall negative experience, with most patients reporting that they received inadequate information about their condition.[2] Thorough understanding of pregnancy-related conditions, their management both in the ED and outpatient setting can allow us to better care for our patients and provide them guidance about their expected course.

Department of Emergency Medicine, Indiana University School of Medicine, 720 Eskenazi Avenue | FOB 3rd Floor, Indianapolis, IN 46202, USA
* Corresponding author.
E-mail address: smanning4@iuhealth.org

Emerg Med Clin N Am 41 (2023) 295–305
https://doi.org/10.1016/j.emc.2022.12.003
0733-8627/23/© 2022 Elsevier Inc. All rights reserved.

emed.theclinics.com

SPONTANEOUS ABORTION

Spontaneous abortion, also referred to as early pregnancy loss or miscarriage, is the loss of an intrauterine pregnancy before the 13th week of gestation. Spontaneous abortion can be further characterized by the stage at which a patient presents for evaluation (**Table 1**). Spontaneous abortion is estimated to affect 13.5% to 16.6% of recognized pregnancies and accounts for the vast majority of pregnancy losses overall.[3–5] The risk of spontaneous abortion increases with maternal age and an increase of 1% to 2% has been observed in all age groups during the past 2 decades.[3] Despite its high incidence, the public still perceives spontaneous abortion as a rare event with respondents in one study estimating its incidence at 5% or less.[6]

Pathophysiology

The pathophysiology of spontaneous abortion remains poorly understood. Spontaneous abortion is likely due to a complex interplay of parental age, genetic, immunologic, hormonal, and environmental factors.[3,4] Chromosomal abnormalities are thought to play a large role in most spontaneous abortions with genetic abnormalities observed in nearly half of all spontaneous abortions.[7] Trisomy and monosomy account for nearly all cases with chromosomes 16, 22, and the sex chromosomes observed most frequently.[7] Maternal age is the strongest maternal risk factor for spontaneous abortion with rates of 8.9% observed in women aged 20 to 24 years and 74.7% in those aged 45 years or older.[8] This association is thought to be primarily due to the higher incidence of genetic abnormalities with advancing maternal age but additional age-related factors include hypertension, type II diabetes, and atherosclerosis.[4] Other conditions associated with increased risk of spontaneous abortion include autoimmune diseases, particularly antiphospholipid syndrome, hematologic diseases, and thyroid disorders, among others.[9,10]

Data regarding euploid spontaneous abortion remains sparce; however, some emerging data suggest that the vaginal microbiota may play a pathophysiologic role. Grewal and colleagues demonstrated that vaginal flora depleted of *Lactobacillus* species are observed more frequently in those who suffer euploid spontaneous abortion versus those with aneuploid spontaneous abortion. Furthermore, authors identified higher levels of proinflammatory cytokines including interleukin (IL)-1β, IL-8, and IL-6 in patients with *Lactobacillus*-depleted vaginal flora suggesting a potential

Table 1 Spontaneous abortion subtypes	
Spontaneous Abortion Subtype	**Definition**
Threatened abortion	Vaginal bleeding, with or without pain with an intrauterine pregnancy identified on ultrasound
Missed abortion (blighted ovum/embryonic demise)	Failure of pregnancy development or death of the embryo/fetus without expulsion of products of conception. Cervical os is typically closed
Incomplete abortion	Passage of a portion of products of conception with some material remaining in the uterus. Cervical os is closed
Septic spontaneous abortion	Incomplete abortion with associated infection
Inevitable abortion	Ongoing passage of products of conception through an open cervical os
Completed abortion	Full expulsion of products of conception

pathophysiologic mechanism.[11] Environmental factors including maternal and fetal drug exposure have variable risk for spontaneous abortion.[12–14] The data regarding common drug exposures including low-to-moderate alcohol consumption, smoking, and high consumption of caffeine remain inconclusive.[15]

Diagnosis

Painful vaginal bleeding is the typical presentation of a spontaneous abortion. Vaginal bleeding in early pregnancy is, however, a nonspecific finding that can be observed in spontaneous abortion, ectopic pregnancy, molar pregnancy, and normal pregnancy. Approximately 500,000 patients present to the ED each year with a complaint of vaginal bleeding in early pregnancy.[16] Although most patients experiencing vaginal bleeding in early pregnancy will ultimately be stable for discharge, some will experience life-threatening hemorrhage. In a study of nearly 500 patients presenting with vaginal bleeding before the 16th week of pregnancy, 4.3% were classified as critical or emergent based on the American Board of Emergency Medicine's patient acuity definitions.[17] These included those with hemorrhage from ruptured ectopic pregnancy in addition to those with hemorrhage from incomplete abortion and septic abortion.

Ultrasound is the diagnostic imaging modality of choice in the evaluation of patients with bleeding in early pregnancy.[18] Emergency physicians should perform or obtain an ultrasound to evaluate for evidence of intrauterine pregnancy, embryonic viability, and retained products of conception. Ultrasound findings may be diagnostic on the index visit or when compared with prior studies if available (**Table 2**). If an intrauterine pregnancy cannot be confidently identified on ultrasonography, patients should undergo serial beta - human chorionic gonadotropin (β-hCG) measurements and imaging to rule out ectopic pregnancy.

Patients in early pregnancy with hemodynamic instability and heavy vaginal bleeding should undergo pelvic examination to facilitate identification and removal of products of conception from the cervical os. The evidence regarding the role of pelvic examination in hemodynamically stable patients with vaginal bleeding in early pregnancy is inconclusive. Some studies have suggested that pelvic examination does not provide additional information in the stable patient with vaginal bleeding in early pregnancy; however, these studies were limited by small sample sizes and low enrollment.[20,21] If patients have an identified intrauterine pregnancy and limited or resolved bleeding, limited evidence suggests that foregoing pelvic examination may be safe.[20] The purpose and utility of a pelvic examination should always be

Table 2 Ultrasound findings diagnostic of pregnancy failure		
Findings on Index Visit		
Crown rump length of >7 mm with no cardiac activity		
Mean gestational sac diameter of 25 mm with no embryo		
Findings on Comparison		
Prior Scan	**Time Elapsed**	**Index Visit**
Gestational sac without a yolk sac	14 + days	No cardiac activity
Gestational sac with a yolk sac	11 + days	No cardiac activity
Cardiac activity at any gestational age	Any time	No cardiac activity

Adapted from: Doubilet PM, Benson CB, Bourne T, et al. Diagnostic criteria for nonviable pregnancy early in the first trimester. *N Engl J Med.* 2013;369(15):1443-1451. doi:10.1056/NEJMra1302417.[19]

discussed with patients including identification of alternate pathologic conditions including sexually transmitted infections, identification of retained foreign bodies, or traumatic injuries.

Treatment

Treatment strategies for spontaneous abortion include expectant, medical, and surgical management. Patients who present with hemodynamic instability, significant hemorrhage, or evidence of septic abortion should undergo urgent surgical management. In otherwise stable patients, expectant, medical, and surgical management have all been demonstrated to be safe and effective and treatment decisions should incorporate patient preference.[22-24] In the setting of desired pregnancy, patients with threatened abortion and those with pregnancy of undetermined viability should undergo expectant management.[18] Rh status should be determined and Rho(D) immune globulin administered to Rh-negative patients.

Expectant Management

Expectant management results in successful expulsion in approximately 80% of patients.[22] Patients diagnosed with incomplete abortion may have higher success rates of expectant management than those with missed abortion. Emergency physicians should advise patients of anticipated symptoms including moderate-to-heavy vaginal bleeding and uterine cramping, as well as the possibility of failed expectant management requiring surgical intervention. They should also provide patients with clear return precautions regarding excessive bleeding and signs and symptoms of infection. Due to the risk of excessive bleeding, expectant management is not advised in the second trimester.[18] Patients should have close follow-up with obstetrics and gynecology to confirm complete expulsion. Follow-up may consist of ultrasound, urine pregnancy tests, or serial β-hCG measurements.[25]

Medical Management

Medical management of spontaneous abortion has some advantages compared with expectant management, including shorter time to expulsion and decreased need for surgical intervention.[23] The safe and effective use of misoprostol-based therapies is well supported in the literature. Vaginal and sublingual administrations are better tolerated than oral administration.[23] Misoprostol is a synthetic prostaglandin E analog that stimulates uterine contractions leading to expulsion of products of conception. Mifepristone, a progesterone antagonist, may improve efficacy when combined with misoprostol but this evidence is mixed and a recent meta-analysis found no additional benefit.[23] Common side effects of misoprostol include uterine cramping, heavy vaginal bleeding, and gastrointestinal distress, such as diarrhea. American College of Obstetrics and Gynecology (ACOG) recommends a single 800 mg intravaginal dose with the possibility of a repeat dose of 800 mg within the following week.[18] Return precautions similar to those undergoing expectant management should be discussed including excessive bleeding and signs and symptoms of infection.

Surgical Management

Surgical evacuation of the uterus is required for those who present with ongoing hemorrhage, hemodynamic instability, or evidence of septic abortion. Certain comorbidities may make the more controlled approach of surgical management preferable including severe anemia, coagulopathy, or cardiovascular disease.[18] Surgical management may take the form of either sharp curettage, vacuum aspiration, or a combination of these approaches. Vacuum aspiration is associated with decreased blood loss, less pain, and shorter procedure duration.[24] Mechanical vacuum aspiration (MVA) may be accomplished with a mechanical aspiration device under local anesthesia with or without procedural sedation. Feasibility of MVA performed by a consulting gynecologist in the ED has been demonstrated to be safe and effective but evidence remains limited.[26,27]

ABORTION
Epidemiology

Despite increasing interest in reliable data on abortion rates, there are significant limitations to data currently available, particularly at the individual level.[28] From 2015 to 2019, the rate of induced abortions was 11.2 to 11.8 per 1000 women aged 15 to 44 years.[29–31] The majority of women seeking abortion are in their twenties, and more than 90% of induced abortions are performed during the first trimester.[29–31] Less than 1% of abortions were performed after 21-week gestation.[30] Most abortions are performed in women who have had a previous live birth, and more than half of women are undergoing abortion for the first time. Approximately three-fourths of abortions are surgical.[31]

Complications of Abortion

Although abortion is a very safe procedure when managed by medical professionals, complications can occur and include incomplete or failed abortion, hemorrhage, septic abortion, and uterine perforation. Estimated complication rates of induced abortion range from 0.1% to 2.1%, with mortality rates less than 1 per 100,000.[31–35] These estimates are, however, hindered by poor follow-up and variability in reporting protocols.[35,36]

An estimated 14 to 15 out of every 100,000 ED visits for women between the ages of 15 and 49 years are related to an abortion complication.[32,33] The average age of the population seeking care is 26 years, and low-income patients, including those with Medicaid, are overrepresented among patients seeking abortion care in the ED. About three-quarters of abortion-related ED visits resulted in discharge from the ED. The majority of visits required observation only.[33,37] Only 1 in 5 abortion-related ED visits results in a major incident, defined as requiring an inpatient stay, blood transfusion, or surgery.[33]

Although complications are rare overall, the most common is incomplete or failed abortion, which accounts for about half of complications. Infection is the second most common complication, accounting for just more than one-quarter of diagnoses. Hemorrhage accounts for 17% of determined complications, and uterine perforation occurs in fewer than 2%.

Incomplete or failed abortion

The term incomplete abortion conventionally refers to a spontaneous abortion in which some products of conception remain in the uterus, as discussed above. However, the term is also applied in the literature to an induced abortion in which not all products are expulsed. A variety of management strategies exist for an incomplete abortion, including expectant management, medical management, or uterine aspiration.[38–40] Expectant management is successful in approximately three-quarters of cases, with the remaining patients requiring either medical or surgical intervention.[41]

Hemorrhage

The rate of hemorrhage from induced abortion varies by source, with most sources reporting rates of less than 2%.[35,37,42–44] Although the rates of hemorrhage from induced abortion are low overall, it is one of the most common causes of death from abortion performed outside the medical setting.[45] Hemorrhage can be due to atony, coagulopathy, or retained tissue, as well as mechanical complications such as uterine perforation or cervical laceration.[46] Epidemiological data on hemorrhage by trimester is complicated by varying definitions of hemorrhage and inaccurate reporting, particularly for medical abortions. Among surgical abortion, those performed by dilation and curettage have been found to have a higher risk of hemorrhage relative to vacuum aspiration.[42]

Septic abortion

One of the most serious complications of abortion is septic abortion. Although septic abortion can occur after either spontaneous or induced abortion, it is most common after induced abortion, particularly when performed outside of the medical setting.[47,48] Bacteria are introduced into the uterus either through instrumentation or from the vaginal vault due to prolonged bleeding. Once in the uterus, bacteria can enter the placental tissue, and ultimately the endometrium.[48] Typically, bacteria responsible for septic abortion are native to vaginal tissue.[48,49] Although a variety of antibiotic regimens have been proposed, the best evidence supports a regimen of ampicillin, gentamicin, and metronidazole as triple therapy.[50,51] **Table 3** shows effectiveness rates of several common regimens.

Uterine perforation

Uncommonly, uterine perforation can occur as a complication of dilation and curettage, although rates are as low as 0.04% to 2.3%.[32,36,37,52–54] Perforation most commonly occurs at the fundus of the uterus, although perforation of the cervix has occasionally been reported.[55] The risk of perforation can be reduced through careful dilation with dilator introduced only a short distance beyond the cervical os. Careful bimanual examination to determine the position and size of the uterus, as well as considering supplementary therapies such as cervical softening with misoprostol before dilation, can help reduce the risk of perforation.[52,53] Experience of the performing physician has also been associated with lower risk of uterine perforation.[56]

Treatment of Complications

Treatment of hemorrhage, whether due to retained tissue or other cause, includes uterine massage, resuscitative measures such as transfusion, and medical management. Medications used both routinely after abortion to reduce bleeding and also to treat hemorrhage include tranexamic acid, misoprostol, methylergonovine maleate, oxytocin, and vasopressin. Bakri balloons serve as a physical barrier to reduce bleeding. In low resource settings, compression devices such as a nonpneumatic

Table 3
Antibiotic regimens for septic abortion[48,50]

Regimen	Success Rate (%)	Notes
Ampicillin, gentamicin, metronidazole	100	Best overall regimen
Pipercillin-tazobactam	93.3	Best single-agent effectiveness
Levofloxacin and metronidazole	86.6	Appropriate in penicillin-allergic patients
Clindamycin and gentamicin	82.2	Appropriate in penicillin-allergic patients

antishock garment may be practical.[57] In the case of retained tissue, both misoprostol and uterine aspiration have high rates of success, with literature reporting both equivalent outcomes and slightly higher success rates for surgical management.[39,40] Unlike septic abortion, there is not adequate evidence to support routine use of antibiotics for incomplete abortion in the absence of signs of infection.[38,58] Although hospital admission is required in cases of septic abortion and uterine perforation with or without visceral injury or intraperitoneal hemorrhage, hemodynamically stable patients with incomplete abortion and controlled hemorrhage may be candidates for observation or urgent outpatient obstetric follow-up.

Changing Regulatory Environment

The regulatory environment for abortion has entered a period of dramatic change within the past 10 years. At the time of writing, the Supreme Court had just issued a landmark decision in *Dobbs vs. Jackson Women's Health Organization*, which overturned *Roe vs. Wade* (1973), the original court decision stating that women had a constitutional right to abortion. With the decision in *Dobbs vs. Jackson*, the legality of abortion returns to the state level, allowing for the regulation of abortion to differ dramatically among US states.

Although *Dobbs vs. Jackson* is novel in allowing states to outlaw abortion entirely, the past decade had already seen an increasing number of restrictions. Nearly one-third of the current laws regulating abortion have been enacted since 2010.[59] Demand-side laws include restrictions such as preabortion waiting periods, mandatory ultrasounds, and parental notification.[60] Supply-side regulations are designed to limit access to abortion, either through limitations on physicians and clinicians who provide abortions, or through laws regarding abortion facilities themselves. Supply-side regulations are commonly known as Targeted Regulation of Abortion Providers (TRAP) laws. TRAP laws have been associated with decreased rates of abortion, raising concerns about restricted access.[61] The proliferation of TRAP laws since 2010 has drawn sharp rebuke from the ACOG, and other major professional medical societies.[62]

With the *Dobbs vs. Jackson* decision, so-called trigger laws, which outlaw abortion entirely rather than placing demand or supply-side regulations on the procedure come into effect. These laws are in place in 13 states, with several more considered likely to ban the procedure. However, 16 states and the District of Columbia explicitly protect the right to abortion. Thus, great variation in the state-level regulatory environment for abortion is likely to persist for years to come.

The increasing restrictions on abortions during the past decade have given way to discussion on how to reduce harm from abortion performed outside the medical setting. These discussions are likely to increase in the current regulatory environment. One proposal is to improve access and education for women to self-administer misoprostol in order to induce abortion in the case of unwanted pregnancy.[59] This harm-reduction strategy could decrease the rate of maternal deaths due to illegal and unsafe abortion, which was at its peak before *Roe*.[63–65] Other proposals include expanding the number of clinicians able to provide abortion and training medical professionals in the management of complications related to unsafe abortions.[62] The role of the emergency physician in such harm-reduction strategies and their impact on emergency medicine practice has yet to be determined.

The changing regulatory environment, as discussed above, has the potential to affect both the frequency of abortion-related ED visits as well as their acuity. Previous study has shown a relationship between state-level abortion restrictions and the incidence of unsafe abortions, as well as the frequency of ED visits related to unsafe abortions. Unsafe abortions may be related to herbal remedies and other nontraditional ingestions, insertion of vaginal foreign bodies, or self-imposed abdominal trauma.[66–68] Thus, as more regulations are placed on abortion, emergency physicians will need to become familiar with complications that were previously less common. Emergency physicians should also familiarize themselves with any local reporting laws regarding ED visits following abortion.

SUMMARY

Spontaneous and complicated therapeutic abortions have a wide range of presentations and management strategies. Emergency physicians must be adept in the timely diagnosis and management of these conditions. A thorough knowledge of the management approaches their anticipated course may allow emergency physicians to provide more competent and compassionate care during a time of both psychological and physiological stress. Emergency physicians should take particular care to familiarize themselves with the management of complicated therapeutic abortion given the risk of increased rates of clandestine abortions particularly in states with no or limited access to legal abortion.

CLINICS CARE POINTS

- Approximately 1 in 5 patients with spontaneous abortion will require either medical or surgical management.
- Pelvic examination should be performed in patients with ongoing hemorrhage or hemodynamic instability to facilitate removal of products of conception from the cervical os.
- Septic abortions are often polymicrobial reflecting common vaginal flora, thus a broad spectrum antibiotic regimen is recommended.
- Emergency physicians should be aware of their local laws regarding abortion complications including reporting requirements.

DISCLOSURE

The authors have nothing to disclose.

REFERENCES

1. Rui P, Kang K. National Hospital Ambulatory Medical Care Survey: 2017 emergency department summary tables. Natl Cent Heal Stat. 2017. Available at: https://www.cdc.gov/nchs/data/nham. Accessed September 16, 2022.
2. Baird S, Gagnon MD, DeFiebre G, et al. Women's experiences with early pregnancy loss in the emergency room: A qualitative study. Sex Reprod Healthc 2018;16(March 2018):113–7.
3. Rossen LM, Ahrens KA, Branum AM. Trends in risk of pregnancy loss among US women, 1990-2011. Paediatr Perinat Epidemiol 2018;32(1):19–29.
4. Magnus MC, Morken N-H, Wensaas K-A, et al. Risk of miscarriage in women with chronic diseases in Norway: a registry linkage study. PLoS Med 2021;18(5):e1003603.
5. Wilcox AJ, Weinberg CR, O'Connor JF, et al. Incidence of early loss of pregnancy. N Engl J Med 1988;319(4):189–94.
6. Bardos J, Hercz D, Friedenthal J, et al. A national survey on public perceptions of miscarriage. Obstet Gynecol 2015;125(6):1313–20.

7. Zhang X, Fan J, Chen Y, et al. Cytogenetic analysis of the products of conception after spontaneous abortion in the first trimester. Cytogenet Genome Res 2021; 161(3–4):120–31.

8. Nybo Andersen AM, Wohlfahrt J, Christens P, et al. Maternal age and fetal loss: population based register linkage study. BMJ 2000;320(7251):1708–12.

9. Chen S, Zhou X, Zhu H, et al. Preconception TSH and pregnancy outcomes: a population-based cohort study in 184 611 women. Clin Endocrinol (Oxf) 2017; 86(6):816–24.

10. Liu X, Chen Y, Ye C, et al. Hereditary thrombophilia and recurrent pregnancy loss: a systematic review and meta-analysis. Hum Reprod 2021;36(5):1213–29.

11. Grewal K, Lee YS, Smith A, et al. Chromosomally normal miscarriage is associated with vaginal dysbiosis and local inflammation. BMC Med 2022;20(1):38.

12. Hoover RN, Hyer M, Pfeiffer RM, et al. Adverse health outcomes in women exposed in utero to diethylstilbestrol. N Engl J Med 2011;365(14):1304–14.

13. Lee H, Koh J-W, Kim Y-A, et al. Pregnancy and neonatal outcomes after exposure to alprazolam in pregnancy. Front Pharmacol 2022;13(April):854562.

14. Lammer EJ, Chen DT, Hoar RM, et al. Retinoic acid embryopathy. N Engl J Med 1985;313(14):837–41.

15. Maconochie N, Doyle P, Prior S, et al. Risk factors for first trimester miscarriage–results from a UK-population-based case-control study. BJOG 2007;114(2): 170–86.

16. Wittels KA, Pelletier AJ, Brown DFM, et al. United States emergency department visits for vaginal bleeding during early pregnancy, 1993-2003. Am J Obstet Gynecol 2008;198(5):523.e1–6.

17. McAllister A, Lang B, Flynn A, et al. Pregnant and bleeding: a model to assess factors associated with the need for emergency care in early pregnancy. Am J Emerg Med 2022;53:94–8.

18. ACOG. ACOG Practice Bulletin No. 200 summary: early pregnancy loss. Obstet Gynecol 2018;132(5):1311–3.

19. Doubilet PM, Benson CB, Bourne T, et al. Diagnostic criteria for nonviable pregnancy early in the first trimester. N Engl J Med 2013;369(15):1443–51.

20. Linden JA, Grimmnitz B, Hagopian L, et al. is the pelvic examination still crucial in patients presenting to the emergency department with vaginal bleeding or abdominal pain when an intrauterine pregnancy is identified on ultrasonography? A randomized controlled trial. Ann Emerg Med 2017;70(6):825–34.

21. Johnstone C. Vaginal examination does not improve diagnostic accuracy in early pregnancy bleeding. EMA - Emerg Med Australas 2013;25(3):219–21.

22. Luise C, Jermy K, May C, et al. Outcome of expectant management of spontaneous first trimester miscarriage: observational study. BMJ 2002;324(7342): 873–5.

23. Lemmers M, Verschoor MAC, Kim BV, et al. Medical treatment for early fetal death (less than 24 weeks). Cochrane Database Syst Rev 2019;6(6):CD002253.

24. Tunçalp O, Gülmezoglu AM, Souza JP. Surgical procedures for evacuating incomplete miscarriage. Cochrane Database Syst Rev 2010;9:CD001993.

25. Grossman D, Grindlay K. Alternatives to ultrasound for follow-up after medication abortion: a systematic review. Contraception 2011;83(6):504–10.

26. Kinariwala M, Quinley KE, Datner EM, et al. Manual vacuum aspiration in the emergency department for management of early pregnancy failure. Am J Emerg Med 2013;31(1):244–7.

27. Whittaker L, Pymar H, Liu X-Q. Manual uterine aspiration in the emergency department as a first-line therapy for early pregnancy loss: a single-centre retrospective study. J Obstet Gynaecol Can 2022;44(6):644–9.
28. Ahrens KA, Hutcheon JA. Time for better access to high-quality abortion data in the United States. Am J Epidemiol 2020;189(7):640–7.
29. Kortsmit K, Jatlaoui TC, Mandel MG, et al. Abortion Surveillance — United States, 2018. MMWR Surveill Summ 2020;69(7):1–30.
30. Kortsmit K, Mandel MG, Reeves JA, et al. Abortion Surveillance — United States, 2019. MMWR Surveill Summ 2021;70(9):1–29.
31. Jatlaoui TC, Boutot ME, Mandel MG, et al. Abortion Surveillance - United States, 2015. MMWR Surveill Summ 2018;67(13):1–45.
32. Orlowski MH, Soares WE, Kerrigan KL, et al. Management of postabortion complications for the emergency medicine clinician. Ann Emerg Med 2021;77(2):221–32.
33. Upadhyay UD, Johns NE, Barron R, et al. Abortion-related emergency department visits in the United States: an analysis of a national emergency department sample. BMC Med 2018;16(1):1–11.
34. Cleland K, Creinin MD, Nucatola D, et al. Significant adverse events and outcomes after medical abortion. Obstet Gynecol 2013;121(1):166–71.
35. Upadhyay UD, Desai S, Zlidar V, et al. Incidence of emergency department visits and complications after abortion. Obstet Gynecol 2015;125(1):175–83.
36. Grossman D, Blanchard K, Blumenthal P. Complications after second trimester surgical and medical abortion. Reprod Health Matters 2008;16(31 SUPPL):173–82.
37. White K, Carroll E, Grossman D. Complications from first-trimester aspiration abortion: a systematic review of the literature. Contraception 2015;92(5):422–38.
38. American College of Obstetricians and Gynecologists' Committee on Practice Bulletins—Gynecology S of FP. Medication Abortion Up to 70 Days of Gestation: ACOG Practice Bulletin, Number 225. Obstet Gynecol 2020;136(4):e31–47.
39. Khaniya B, Yadav R. Comparison of use of misoprostol versus manual vacuum aspiration in the treatment of incomplete abortion. Nepal Med J 2019;2(2):239–42.
40. Ibiyemi KF, Ijaiya MA, Adesina KT. Randomised trial of oral misoprostol versus manual vacuum aspiration for the treatment of incomplete abortion at a nigerian tertiary hospital. Sultan Qaboos Univ Med J 2019;19(1):e38–43.
41. Lemmers M, Verschoor MAC, Oude Rengerink K, et al. MisoREST: Surgical versus expectant management in women with an incomplete evacuation of the uterus after misoprostol treatment for miscarriage: a randomized controlled trial. Hum Reprod 2016;31(11):2421–7.
42. Pestvenidze E, Lomia N, Berdzuli N, et al. Effects of gestational age and the mode of surgical abortion on postabortion hemorrhage and fever: Evidence from population-based reproductive health survey in Georgia. BMC Womens Health 2017;17(1):1–7.
43. Whitehouse K, Fontanilla T, Kim L, et al. Use of medications to decrease bleeding during surgical abortion: a survey of abortion providers' practices in the United States. Contraception 2018;97(6):500–3.
44. Mark KS, Bragg B, Talaie T, et al. Risk of complication during surgical abortion in obese women. Am J Obstet Gynecol 2018;218(2):238.e1–5.
45. Haddad LB, Nour NM. Unsafe abortion: unnecessary maternal mortality. Rev Obstet Gynecol 2009;2(2):122–6.
46. Kerns J, Steinauer J. Management of postabortion hemorrhage. Contraception 2013;87(3):331–42.
47. Stubblefield PG, Grimes DA. Septic abortion. N Engl J Med 1994;331(5):310–4.

48. Eschenbach DA. Treating spontaneous and induced septic abortions. Obstet Gynecol 2015;125(5):1042–8.
49. Rotheram EB, Schick SF. Nonclostridial anaerobic bacteria in septic abortion. Am J Med 1969;46(1):80–9.
50. Fouks Y, Samueloff O, Levin I, et al. Assessing the effectiveness of empiric antimicrobial regimens in cases of septic/infected abortions. Am J Emerg Med 2020; 38(6):1123–8.
51. Udoh A, Effa EE, Oduwole O, et al. Antibiotics for treating septic abortion. Cochrane Database Syst Rev 2015;2015(2). https://doi.org/10.1002/14651858. CD011528.
52. Amarin ZO, Badria LF. A survey of uterine perforation following dilatation and curettage or evacuation of retained products of conception. Arch Gynecol Obstet 2005;271(3):203–6.
53. Chen LH, Lai SF, Lee WH, et al. Uterine perforation during elective first trimester abortions: a 13-year review. Singapore Med J 1995;36(1):63–7.
54. Kaali S, Szigetvari I, Bartfai G. The frequency and management of uterine perforations during first-trimester abortions. Am J Obstet Gynecol 1989;161:406–8.
55. Hefler L, Lemach A, Seebacher V, et al. The intraoperative complication rate of nonobstetric dilation and curettage. Obstet Gynecol 2009;113(6):1268–71.
56. Grimes DA, Schulz KF, Cates WJ. Prevention of uterine perforation during curettage abortion. JAMA J Am Med Assoc 1984;251(16):2108–11.
57. Manandhar S, El Ayadi AM, Butrick E, et al. The role of the nonpneumatic antishock garment in reducing blood loss and mortality associated with postabortion hemorrhage. Stud Fam Plann 2015;46(3):281–96.
58. May W, Gülmezoglu AM, Ba-Thike K. Antibiotics for incomplete abortion. Cochrane Database Syst Rev 2007;4. https://doi.org/10.1002/14651858. CD001779.pub2.
59. Tasset J, Harris LH. Harm reduction for abortion in the United States. Obstet Gynecol 2018;131(4):621–4.
60. Austin N, Harper S. Assessing the impact of TRAP laws on abortion and women's health in the USA: A systematic review. BMJ Sex Reprod Heal 2018;44(2): 128–34.
61. Brown BP, Hebert LE, Gilliam M, et al. Association of Highly Restrictive State Abortion Policies With Abortion Rates, 2000-2014. JAMA Netw Open 2020; 3(11):e2024610.
62. American College of Obstetricians and Gynecologists' Committee on Health Care for Underserved Women AC of O and GAA and TEWG. Increasing Access to Abortion: ACOG Committee Opinion, Number 815. Obstet Gynecol 2020; 136(6):e107–15.
63. Minkoff H, Gibbs RS. Preparing for a post-Roe world. Am J Obstet Gynecol 2019; 220(3):249.e1–3.
64. Harris D, O'Hare D, Pakter J, et al. Legal abortion 1970-1971–the New York City experience. Am J Public Health 1973;63(5):409–18.
65. Guttmacher A. Induced abortion. New York J Med 1963;63:2334.
66. Conway GA, Slocumb JC. Plants used as abortifacients and emmenagogues by Spanish New Mexicans. J Ethnopharmacol 1979;1(3):241–61.
67. Honigman B, Davila G, Petersen J. Reemergence of self-induced abortions. J Emerg Med 1993;11(1):105–12.
68. Harris LH, Grossman D. Complications of Unsafe and Self-Managed Abortion. N Engl J Med 2020;382(11):1029–40.

Management of Coronavirus Disease-2019 Infection in Pregnancy

Vivian Lam, MD, MPH[a], Kami M. Hu, MD, FAAEM FACEP[a,b,*]

KEYWORDS

- COVID-19 • SARS-COV-2 • Pregnancy • Antepartum • Obstetrics

KEY POINTS

- Pregnancy is inherently associated with an increased risk of severe illness and poor fetal outcomes related to coronavirus disease-2019 (COVID-19) infection.
- Although evidence for the management of pregnant patients with COVID-19 infection is limited, all major guidelines argue against the withholding of therapeutics solely due to pregnancy.
- Oxygenation goals in pregnancy are higher (saturations $\geq$ 95% or $PaO_2 > 70$ mm Hg), leading to the achievement of "severe illness" status and the need for adjustments to therapeutic decisions earlier than nonpregnant counterparts with COVID-19 infection.
- The basic tenets of COVID-19-related acute respiratory distress syndrome and critical illness management are largely the same for pregnant patients as in nonpregnant patients, with exception of oxygenation goals, lower recommended PCO_2 ranges, and a need for fetal monitoring.
- Pregnancy is not a contraindication to extracorporeal membrane oxygenation (ECMO) cannulation. Referral to an ECMO-capable institution should be considered for pregnant patients with refractory hypoxia despite maximum therapy.

INTRODUCTION

The coronavirus disease-2019 (COVID-19) pandemic has had far-reaching impacts on the provision of health care to many populations. As providers learned in real-time how to care for all-comers with COVID-19 infection, there came the realization that pregnancy is associated with more severe illness and poor maternal and fetal outcomes. In this light, navigating the literature to determine the appropriate care has been particularly important for physicians caring for pregnant women.

[a] Department of Internal Medicine, Section of Critical Care Medicine, Advocate Christ Medical Center, 4440 West 95th Street, Suite AIP, Oak Lawn, IL 60453, USA; [b] Division of Pulmonary & Critical Care, Department of Internal Medicine, University of Maryland, School of Medicine, 110 South Paca Street, 6th Floor Suite 200, Baltimore, MD 21201, USA
* Corresponding author. Department of Emergency Medicine, Department of Internal Medicine, Division of Pulmonary & Critical Care, University of Maryland, School of Medicine, 110 South Paca Street, 6th Floor Suite 200, Baltimore, MD 21201, USA.
E-mail address: khu@som.umaryland.edu
Twitter: @kwhomd (K.M.H.)

Emerg Med Clin N Am 41 (2023) 307–322
https://doi.org/10.1016/j.emc.2022.12.004
0733-8627/23/© 2023 Elsevier Inc. All rights reserved.
emed.theclinics.com

Epidemiologically, the data suggest that pregnant patients have similar positive test rates to the general local population,[1] and that the majority of pregnant patients with COVID-19 infection experience mild disease.[2] In comparison to their nonpregnant age-matched counterparts; however, pregnant patients have an increased risk of severe illness including intensive care unit (ICU) admission and need for mechanical ventilation and extracorporeal membrane oxygenation (ECMO) support.[1,3,4] Similarly, pregnant patients with COVID-19 have a higher incidence of poor fetal and neonatal outcomes and death than noninfected pregnant patients.[1]

Several groups have provided recommendations for the care of pregnant patients during the COVID pandemic,[5–8] relying on general population data, animal safety studies, and expert opinion. One important overarching theme is clear across them: therapy needed for the management of COVID-19 should not be withheld solely based on pregnancy.

EVALUATION

The level of the diagnostic evaluation in pregnant patients presenting with a viral syndrome suspicious of COVID-19 is essentially the same as for nonpregnant patients and depends on their apparent illness severity and baseline comorbidities. Patients with mild flu-like illness may only need testing to evaluate for flu and COVID, for example, whereas symptoms of *per os* intolerance and diarrhea may require bloodwork, and critical illness requires much more.

Specific considerations in pregnant individuals include the determination of fetal well-being. This evaluation includes asking about abdominal cramping, leakage of vaginal fluid or vaginal bleeding, and presence of fetal movement if gestational age-appropriate, and performing a point-of-care-ultrasound (POCUS) assessment of fetal heart rate. Appropriate chest imaging should not be avoided if indicated, as the radiation exposure is relatively low,[9] and presence of infiltrates inform further care. Finally, evaluation for exertional hypoxia is necessary for any pregnant individual with moderate COVID-19 infection without evident hypoxia at rest.

CLASSIFICATION OF DISEASE SEVERITY

Management of COVID-19 infection is primarily dependent on illness severity. The range of clinical presentation of COVID-19 infection is wide and the definition of illness categories may vary slightly across clinical guidelines and studies. This article uses the definitions as delineated in the National Institutes of Health (NIH) guidelines,[7] **(Table 1)** which are generally accepted by the Society for Maternal-Fetal Medicine (SMFM).[5]

(Placeholder: see **Table 1**. COVID-19 Infection Severity Classification[7]).

Coronavirus Disease-2019 Therapeutics

This article will briefly discuss pharmacologic therapies currently recommended by major societies and panels, which are summarized in **Tables 2** and **3**. Pregnancy remains an independent risk factor for progression to severe disease and adverse outcomes, and both the American College of Obstetricians and Gynecologists (ACOG) and the Society for Maternal-Fetal Medicine (SMFM) have been explicit in their statements that appropriate therapies should not be withheld from pregnant patients.[5,6]

(Placeholder: **Table 2**. Recommended therapies for COVID-19 management).

Antivirals

Nirmatrelvir/ritonavir (paxlovid)
Recommended for the management of symptomatic outpatients with a risk of progression to severe disease,[10] ritonavir-boosted nimatrelvir decreases the risk of

Table 1	
Coronavirus disease-2019 infection severity classification	
Severity Class	**Presentation**
Asymptomatic Or Presymptomatic	Positive COVID-19 test without symptoms
Mild	Flu-like symptoms (ex: fever, cough, sore throat, vomiting, diarrhea, malaise) No dyspnea or hypoxia and normal chest imaging
Moderate	Evidence of lower respiratory tract disease by symptoms or imaging $SpO_2 \geq 95\%$ on room air
Severe	Respiratory rate > 30 breaths/minute Hypoxia with $SpO_2 < 95\%$ on room air PaO_2 to FiO_2 ratio < 300 Lung involvement on imaging > 50%
Critical	Multisystem organ dysfunction Circulatory shock Respiratory failure requiring HFNC or MV

Abbreviations: FiO_2, fraction of inspired oxygen; HFNC, high flow nasal cannula; MV, mechanical ventilation (invasive or noninvasive); PaO_2, arterial partial pressure of oxygen; SpO_2, oxygen saturation.

hospitalization and mortality in COVID-19 infection.[11] Though the EPIC-HR trial supporting its use excluded pregnant and lactating individuals, the combo is still recommended for patients in this category who are pregnant,[5,7] based on an assessment of the low risk of harm given existing animal safety data[12] and small case series.[13]

Remdesivir

Remdesivir was one of the earliest antivirals available for the management of COVID-19, used in hospitalized patients in the ACTT-1 trial with earlier disease recovery.[14] Remdesivir has also been studied in outpatients at high risk of progression to reduce the risk of hospitalization and death.[15]

In pregnancy specifically, evidence regarding the use of remdesivir to treat COVID-19 is accumulating but is primarily observational. A small study suggested that early administration of remdesivir (within seven days of symptom onset) is associated with a decreased likelihood of progression to critical disease or ICU admission as well as decreased length of hospitalization.[16] A case series of pregnant individuals described clinical improvement and no adverse events after remdesivir,[17] and a recent systematic review noted a high rate of recovery among remdesivir-treated pregnant patients, significantly higher than those not treated.[18] Better outcomes were seen in patients with better baseline health and drug administration within 48 hours of presentation.[18]

Animal reproductive studies have not shown adverse fetal effects,[19] and prior use in the treatment of Ebola-infected pregnant individuals also support its safety.[20] The most demonstrated adverse event is transaminitis, with higher levels seen with 10-day versus 5-day treatment regimens. These lab abnormalities have not resulted in poor clinical outcomes and eventually resolve on cessation of the drug,[18] making it quite reasonable to use remdesivir for a planned 5-day course, with the determination to continue to 10 days if deemed necessary.

Molnupiravir

Molnupiravir is another second-line antiviral therapy with lower efficacy and no human pregnancy data. Although the FDA and WHO recommend against its use in pregnancy due to teratogenicity noted in animal studies,[21] the NIH panel suggests that molnupiravir can be a reasonable last option for pregnant patients at particularly high risk of

Table 2
Recommended therapies for coronavirus disease-2019 management

Drug Class	Name	Indication	Dose	Side Effects	Pregnancy Consideration
Antivirals	Nirmatrelvir/Ritonavir (Paxlovid)	Outpatients with mild/moderate severity at high risk for severe illness ≤5 days onset	Nirmatrelvir 300 mg/RTV 100 mg twice daily for 5 days eGFR ≥30 to 60 mL/min: Nirmatrelvir 150 mg/RTV 100 mg twice daily for 5 days	• GI effects • Hypertension • Myalgias • Angioedema; hypersensitivity reactions	Nirmatrelvir: no safety data RTV considered safe Not recommended by WHO
	Remdesivir	Mild/moderate severity at high risk for severe illness Severe illness not on MV/ECMO ≤7 days onset	200 mg IV on day 1, then IV daily Mild/moderate: 3 days Severe: 5-10 days	No increase from placebo	Considered safe Requires multiple IV doses
	Molnupiravir	Outpatients with mild/moderate severity at high risk for severe illness ≤5 days onset	800 mg twice daily for 5 days	No increase from placebo	NIH/SMFM: last option if other therapies unavailable Not recommended by WHO or FDA
Monoclonal Antibodies	Tixagevimab/Cilgavimab (Evusheld) Casirivimab/Imdevimab (REGEN-COV) Sotrovimab Bebtelovimab	Outpatients with mild/moderate severity at high risk for severe illness ≤7 days onset Not currently recommended for treatment given low efficacy against circulating variants	175 mg IV over 30 seconds	Hypersensitivity reactions No increase from placebo	2nd line therapy Limited data Generally considered safe

Steroids	Dexamethasone	Severe/critical illness	6 mg daily for 10 days ARDS: 20 mg IV daily x 5 days then 10 mg daily x 5 days	Hyperglycemia	Dexamethasone crosses the placenta, risk of neonatal adrenal insufficiency depending on duration/timing of delivery
JAK Inhibitors	Baricitinib	Severe/critical illness ≤ 7 days onset	4 mg PO daily for 14 days or until hospital discharge eGFR 30-59: 2 mg daily eGFR 15-29: 1 mg daily eGFR <15: not for use	• No increase from placebo • Cytopenias • Transaminitis • Thrombosis	No safety data
	Tofacitinib	Severe/critical illness with baricitinib unavailable (no set limit)	10 mg twice daily for 14 days or until hospital discharge eGFR <30: 5 mg twice daily ESRD: 5 mg twice daily, give dose after HD on HD days	• Thrombosis • Cardiovascular events • GI perforation	No evidence of fetal adverse effects Must use with VTE prophylaxis
IL-6 Receptor Antagonists	Tocilizumab	Severe/critical illness	8 mg/kg IV once (maximum dose 800 mg)	• Transaminitis • Activation of latent infection	Animal studies with evidence of fetal toxicity at high doses Appears safe in COVID-19
	Sarilumab	Severe/critical illness with tocilizumab unavailable	400 mg IV once	• Cytopenias • Transaminitis • Activation of latent infection	No human safety data Appears safe in animals

Abbreviations: ECMO, extracorporeal membrane oxygenation; eGFR, estimated glomerular filtration rate; FDA, Federal Drug Administration; GI, gastrointestinal; HD, hemodialysis; IL-6, interleukin-6; IV, intravenous; JAK, Janus kinase; kg, kilogram; mg, milligram; mL/min, milliliter per minute; NIH, National Institutes of Health; RTV, ritonavir; SMFM, Society of Maternal Fetal Medicine; WHO, World Health Organization.

Data from [National Institutes of Health COVID-19 Treatment Guidelines Panel. Clinical Management of Adults. Updated 26 Sept 2022. Available at: https://www.covid19treatmentguidelines.nih.gov/management/clinical-management-of-adults/. Accessed 22 Nov 2022.] *and* [Society for Maternal-Fetal Medicine. COVID-19 Outpatient Therapy for Pregnant Patients. Updated 21 Jun 2022. Available at: chrome-extension://efaidnbmnnnibpcajpcglclefindmkaj/https://s3.amazonaws.com/cdn.smfm.org/media/3526/COVID_treatment_table_6-21-22_%28final%29.pdf. Accessed 22 Nov 2022.]

Table 3
Major recommendations for coronavirus disease-2019 therapy based on severity of illness[5,8,10,31]

| Illness | Major Guidelines | | |
Severity	WHO	NIH/SMFM[a]	IDSA
Asymptomatic			
Mild	High risk: Remdesivir	High risk, not hospitalized:	Not hospitalized: Remdesivir
Moderate	Avoid Nirmatrelvir/Ritonavir and Molnupiravir[b]	Preferred 1st: Nirmatrelvir/Ritonavir 2nd: Remdesivir Alternative: Molnupiravir Hospitalized: Remdesivir	Can consider convalescent plasma if immunosuppressed High risk: Add Nirmatrelvir/Ritonavir (not Molnupiravir)[b] Hospitalized: Remdesivir
Severe	Dexamethasone AND Tocilizumab (2nd: Sarilumab) AND Baricitinib Consider addition of Remdesivir	"Minimal" O2: Remdesivir Conventional O2: Remdesivir AND Dexamethasone Rapid progression/Systemic inflammation[c]: Add Baricitinib or Tocilizumab	Dexamethasone AND Remdesivir AND Baricitinib (2nd: Tofacitinib) Rapid progression/Systemic inflammation[c]: Add Tocilizumab (2nd: Sarilumab)
Critical	Dexamethasone AND Tocilizumab (2nd: Sarilumab) AND Baricitinib	Dexamethasone AND Baricitinib (2nd line: Tofacitinib) OR Tocilizumab (2nd line: Sarilumab) If not yet requiring MV or ECMO: can add Remdesivir	Dexamethasone AND Tocilizumab (or 2nd: Sarilumab)

Abbreviations: NIH, National Institutes of Health COVID-19 Treatment Guidelines; WHO, World Health Organization; SMFM, Society for Maternal Fetal Medicine.
[a] Follows NIH Clinical Guidelines.
[b] Pregnancy-specific recommendation.
[c] C-reactive protein >75 mg/L.

severe disease unable to receive other therapies, especially during later gestation after embryogenesis.[7]

Monoclonal Antibodies

A variety of severe acute respiratory syndrome coronavirus 2 (SARS-COV-2)-targeting monoclonal antibodies are available for use to prevent the progression of COVID-19 disease severity. Bebtelovimab was the last available antibody under an emergency use authorization (EUA) by the FDA for use in the treatment of COVID-19, but this EUA was rescinded in November 2022 due to lack of efficacy against circulating variants. Tixagevimab/cilgavimab (brand name Evusheld) is under FDA EUA for pre-exposure prophylaxis but not therapy. Of note, European Union's European Medicines Agency supports the use of tixagevimbab/cilgavimab in treatment, due to some existing evidence of its efficacy.[22,23] Diminished efficacy against the newer variants has led to the FDA removing its EUA for the use of casirivimab/imdevimab (REGEN-COV), sotrovimab, and bamlanivimab/etesevimab at this time.[24]

The actual data on bebtelovimab use in pregnancy are limited, with existing literature on monoclonal antibody efficacy and safety in pregnant women generally including the earlier generation antibodies. These studies are primarily retrospective in nature but support clinical efficacy in preventing the progression to severe COVID-19 infection.[25–29] Hypersensitivity reactions, including anaphylaxis, have occurred and remain a risk with monoclonal antibody administration, and one case series reported a subsequent early delivery necessitated by fetal distress,[29] but with this singular exception, the safety profile appears to be relatively favorable.[30]

Immunomodulators

Janus kinase inhibitors (baricitinib and tofacitinib)
Many immunomodulatory drugs have been evaluated for the management of COVID-19. The Janus kinase (JAK) inhibitors baricitinib and tofacitinib are currently recommended by the Infectious Disease Society of America (IDSA) for the treatment of severely to critically ill patients with COVID-19 infection,[31] with a stronger recommendation for baricitinib based on multiple trials in nonpregnant patients indicating decreased need for mechanical ventilation and 60-day mortality, whether used alone or in conjunction with dexamethasone or remdesivir.[32,33] The data for tofacitinib is less robust, but its use was associated with reduced incidence of death or progressive respiratory failure when given in conjunction with dexamethasone.[34]

Although no differences in rates of adverse events were seen in the COVID-19 studies, both drugs have been associated with increased thrombotic risk,[35] a factor of potential concern given the existing increased risk of venous thromboembolism (VTE) in pregnancy. This risk should be considered in the context of JAK inhibitors' potential to reduce both progression to respiratory failure that leads to lengthy immobility as well as the systemic inflammation which is presumed to lead to thrombotic risk in COVID-19 infection. All pregnant patients hospitalized due to COVID-19 infection should receive pharmacologic VTE prophylaxis unless specifically contraindicated.[5,6] Although limited, the existing literature does not support an increased frequency of poor fetal outcomes with maternal baricitinib or tofacitinib use in other autoimmune disorders.[36–38]

Interleukin-6 inhibitors (tocilizumab and sarilumab)
Tocilizumab is the primary interleukin-6 (IL-6) receptor antagonist currently recommended for use.[5–8,31] Used in conjunction with corticosteroids in the treatment of severe to critically ill COVID-19 infection and systemic inflammation (widely defined as a C-reactive protein level >75 mg/L), it has been associated with lower mortality,

decrease in progression to mechanical ventilation, and earlier discharge in the general population.[39,40] The only randomized controlled data in pregnant COVID-19 infection arises from the RECOVERY study, which included 10 pregnant patients.[39]

Clinical safety data for tocilizumab use during pregnancy exist to a small degree in the rheumatologic disease literature.[41,42] There is evidence of higher prematurity and spontaneous abortion rates, but these findings are confounded by concomitant methotrexate use–a known abortifacient–and disease activity in the rheumatologic population. In the limited data from the current pandemic[43–45] there is no evidence of increased congenital malformation risk, although infection has been a continuing concern. One study noted a single CMV reactivation and subsequent congenital CMV,[43] and UK guidelines suggest delay of live vaccines until 6 months of age in case of in utero exposure to tocilizumab.[44]

Corticosteroids

The primary standard medical management of COVID-19 of this severity includes corticosteroids for pregnant patients with saturations of <95% on room air.[46] The RECOVERY trial demonstrating survival benefit with dexamethasone only included 4 pregnant patients,[46] but the marked benefits led to the recommendation that COVID-infected pregnant patients with an oxygen requirement be given steroids according to RECOVERY dosing (6 mg daily for 10 days).[5] In the case that steroids are indicated for fetal lung maturity (<34 weeks), the SMFM recommends dosing of dexamethasone 6 mg IM every 12 h for 48 h before the 6 mg daily dosing for up to 10 days.[5]

Almost coincident with the beginning of the COVID-19 pandemic, the DEXA-ARDS trial was published, adding to the many previous trials with conflicting data regarding steroids in ARDS. DEXA-ARDS demonstrated increased ventilator-free days and decreased mortality among ARDS patients with P:F ratio <200 using a treatment regimen of 20 mg dexamethasone daily for 5 days followed by 10 mg daily for 5 days, without significant adverse effects.[47] With RECOVERY ushering in dexamethasone as a standard treatment for COVID-19 infection, consideration of high-dose dexamethasone for COVID-19-related ARDS seemed natural. In truth, the optimal steroid dose is unclear despite additional signals for benefit in several studies,[48–50] although additional randomized controlled trials are ongoing. Of note, high-dose dexamethasone is not mentioned in guidelines for pregnant individuals with more severe COVID-19 infection.[5]

(Placeholder: **Table 3**. Recommendations for COVID-19 therapy based on severity of illness).

MANAGEMENT
Asymptomatic Infection

Pregnant patients with asymptomatic COVID-19 infection, in general, require only maintenance of prenatal and follow-up care. The American College of Obstetricians and Gynecologists (ACOG) has developed recommendations regarding use of telehealth and modification or consolidation of routine prenatal care as necessary to limit exposure to others.[6] Therapies to prevent progression of illness (see **Table 2**) should be strongly considered in all pregnant patients and more so in those with additional risk factors placing them at risk for severe illness. Patients should be advised to follow up closely with their outpatient physician and told when to seek care in case of disease progression.[5,6]

Mild/Moderate Disease

Mild disease involves viral syndromic symptoms without dyspnea, hypoxia, or evidence of lower respiratory tract infection by imaging, whereas moderate disease describes individuals with evidence of lower respiratory disease but without oxygen requirement.

An understanding of oxygenation goals in pregnancy is key to appropriately classify disease severity and therefore management of COVID-19 infections. Goal saturations are higher in pregnant patients due to increased oxygen consumption and occurrence of fetal hypoxia and distress at maternal PaO2 values < 60 mm Hg.[51] In vivo data establishing a PaO2 threshold is limited, but current guidelines continue to recommend a goal saturation of ≥95%, corresponding to a PaO2 ≥70 mm Hg.[5] Although nonpregnant patients would be classified as having a moderate disease with saturations of 94%, in pregnancy this qualifies as severe.

Supportive care

In general, the usual symptomatic management of a viral syndrome can and should be provided: acetaminophen for pain and fever control, increased hydration, and short-term over-the-counter (OTC) decongestants as needed are suitable. Guaifenesin and dextromethorphan are considered safe in pregnancy, as are antihistamines. There are no human studies evaluating the use of phenol throat sprays, but some evidence of fetal toxicity in mice studies,[52] leading to a recommendation to use for only short durations and to gargle and spit rather than swallow the spray.

Coronavirus Disease-specific therapies

Most pregnant patients with COVID-19 infection experience mild illness.[2] Although pregnancy is a standalone risk factor for progression to severe infection, many patients and their physicians may opt to defer specific COVID therapies when the illness is asymptomatic or mild. Emergency physicians should maintain a low threshold to treat those with mild illness but a separate additional risk factor for severe illness, as well as those with the moderate disease even if hospitalization is not required.

Disposition

Low-risk pregnant patients with mild COVID-19 infection can usually be discharged home with appropriate guidance on outpatient follow-up with their obstetrician, appropriate supportive care, and indications for prompt return to the ED. The disposition of patients with lower respiratory disease depends primarily on their overall clinical picture, baseline health, ambulatory status, and ability to care for themselves appropriately at home. Patients with moderate illness may be discharged if they do not experience significant exertional dyspnea and their saturations remain ≥95% on ambulation, if they are able to maintain good oral hydration, and if they have an adequate outpatient follow-up. Otherwise, retention in the hospital for further observation and management is appropriate. Patients requiring hospitalization should be admitted to a facility that can conduct fetal monitoring and provide appropriate obstetric or maternal-fetal medicine consultation if indicated by gestational age and patient-specific risk factors.

Severe Disease

Severe disease is defined as COVID-19 infection with hypoxia requiring supplemental oxygen but not high flow nasal cannula (HFNC) or mechanical ventilation (MV), PaO2/FiO2 ratio < 300, respiratory rate >30 breaths per minute, or >50% lung involvement on imaging.

Coronavirus Disease-specific therapies

Administration of steroids is part of the standard of care for all pregnant patients with COVID-19 infection and an oxygen requirement,[31] with a recommendation to administer in conjunction with remdesivir if within 7 days of symptom onset.[5,10,31] It is worth noting that the current NIH guidelines recommend remdesivir alone without dexamethasone for general patients with a new but "minimal" oxygen requirement,[10] but this recommendation is not held across all societies and dexamethasone also potentially be indicated for fetal lung maturation depending on the clinical scenario and gestational age.

Current guidelines also recommend initiation of either baricitinib or tocilizumab in patients with rapidly increasing oxygenation needs or laboratory markers demonstrating systemic inflammation.[10,31] Emergency physicians can usually defer this decision to the admitting team or until consultation with pharmacy or the infectious disease specialists can be performed.

Additional considerations

As already discussed, supplemental oxygenation should be given to reach a goal saturation of $\geq$95%. Proning has been associated with improved oxygenation and decreased mortality in intubated patients with severe acute respiratory distress syndrome (ARDS).[53] Similarly, self-proning arose as a therapeutic adjunct early in the COVID-19 pandemic and is a relatively simple intervention that has been proven to increase oxygenation in patients with severe COVID-19,[54–56] but has not been shown to decrease rates of intubation[57] and can be difficult to manage with the gravid abdomen as pregnancy progresses. If the patient is comfortable doing so, it is reasonable to have them rotate through side-lying positions with pillow support or to prone with use of a pregnancy proning pillow,[5] but escalation to needed respiratory supports should not be delayed to see if self-proning will help.

Disposition

Pregnant patients with hypoxia will, of course, require admission. Owing to the risk of fetal distress with maternal hypoxia and need for quick intervention with decompensation, pregnant patients who have reached fetal viability and have the severe disease should be hospitalized in a facility with ready obstetric and neonatal intensive care capability.

Critical Disease

Critical disease describes the requirement of advanced respiratory therapies including HFNC, noninvasive ventilation (NIV), invasive mechanical ventilation (IMV), or ECMO, as well as patients with shock or other organ dysfunction.

Airway and breathing

The physiologic changes of pregnancy result in a decreased functional reserve with increased oxygen demand; prompt respiratory support to achieve saturations $\geq$95% is crucial to avoid fetal distress and poor outcomes. HFNC has previously been associated with a reduced rate of intubation and ICU mortality compared with NIV in general populations of acute respiratory failure.[58] In COVID-19 infection, there are limited data regarding the selection of HFNC compared with NIV. Guidelines suggest initial management with HFNC in COVID-19 infection with acute hypoxemic respiratory failure despite conventional oxygen therapy,[10] although bypassing HFNC for a trial of NIV may be appropriate depending on the patient's mental status, work of breathing, and concern for poor ventilation. No specific recommendations are available for timing of intubation for COVID-19 during pregnancy and must be considered on a case-by-case basis,[5] although delays to needed intubation have been associated with poor outcomes in patients with both COVID[59] and non-COVID respiratory failure.[60,61]

Special considerations in the pregnant population should inform the preparation for endotracheal intubation. The most experienced practitioner should intubate given aforementioned physiologic changes and needs, including reduced functional residual capacity, increased risk of severe hypoxemia and aspiration, likelihood of a more difficult airway and the need to maintain higher maternal oxygen saturation for adequate fetal oxygenation.[51] If the fetus is viable, in addition to standard fetal heart rate and tocodynamometer monitoring, obstetric and neonatal teams should be present or imminently available, if possible, in case of fetal distress necessitating emergent delivery. Although mechanical ventilation alone is not an indication for delivery, the peri-intubation period presents a time of high risk.

Ventilator management in COVID-19-associated acute respiratory failure should follow the standard guidelines for ventilator management in ARDS. In patients with moderate-severe ARDS, guidelines support a higher PEEP strategy, though this must be assessed based on patient-specific factors some heterogeneity in respiratory failure in COVID-19 patients.[10] With gravid habitus and upward shifting of the diaphragm, a higher PEEP strategy is likely to be beneficial, though there is no formal evidence to support the theory. Minute ventilation is increased in pregnancy, resulting in an average PCO_2 of approximately 30 mm Hg and the necessary maternal-fetal gradient to assist in offloading fetal CO_2 into the maternal circulation to avoid fetal acidemia. Permissive hypercapnia is a major tenet of lung protective ventilation, but there are no formal studies assessing appropriate PCO_2 goals in pregnant ARDS, although values up to 60 mm Hg seems to be reasonably tolerated.[62]

Patients with acute ARDS frequently require sedation and sometimes neuromuscular blockade to tolerate the ventilator settings necessary to improve oxygenation and longer-term outcomes.[63] Deep sedation has been associated with worsened mortality and prolonged mechanical ventilation and hospital length of stay,[64,65] and should *not* be empirically targeted in all patients, but if needed should not be withheld due to concerns of fetal effects.

Circulation
Critical COVID-19 infection can be associated with circulatory shock, whether distributive due to overwhelming systemic inflammation, acidemia, bacterial superinfection, and/or the need to counteract sedative medications that allow ventilator synchrony, or cardiogenic due to myocarditis, or stress-induced versus underlying peripartum cardiomyopathy. Although a fluid restrictive strategy is better for ARDS management,[66] it is important to restore perfusion to the organs, and a 1 or 2-liter bolus of crystalloid is a reasonable initial strategy in light of insensible losses and potential for decreased oral intake or viral gastroenteritis, provided there is no initial concern for cardiogenic shock by physical exam or point-of-care echocardiogram ("echo"). If hypotension persists and patient is volume replete, initiation of vasopressors should be pursued over the additional fluid challenge. Hypotensive patients with signs of volume overload and/or cool extremities and evidence of diminished cardiac function by point-of-care echo should be initiated on inotropic therapy.

Coronavirus Disease-specific therapies
Whether RECOVERY or DEXA-ARDS doses, dexamethasone or an equivalent glucocorticoid, in combination with either baricitinib and/or tocilizumab, are recommended in critically ill patients with COVID-19 infection. see **Table 3**).

Salvage therapy
Critical illness and mechanical ventilation are not specific indications for early delivery, but in patients with severe respiratory failure refractory to maximum therapy beyond 32 weeks gestation, controlled delivery should be considered. After 32 weeks, neonatal major morbidity and mortality are low (8.7% and 0.2%, respectively) with continued decrease as fetal gestational age progresses.[67] Low-level data suggest physiologic improvements in respiratory mechanics in some patients after delivery, although exactly why some benefit and others do not is unclear.[68,69] Delivery could be considered a reasonable option for optimization of both maternal and fetal/neonatal outcomes,

especially in refractory hypoxia and multisystem organ failure, where the risk of decompensation and maternal and fetal mortality is high.

ECMO should be considered as a rescue strategy in pregnant patients with COVID-19 ARDS and refractory hypoxia (PaO_2 <70 mm Hg or $PaO_2:FiO_2$ ratio <150) or hypercapnia (pH < 7.2 or PCO_2 > 80 mm Hg for >6 hours) despite optimal ventilatory management.[5] ECMO cannulation is not in and of itself an indication for delivery, although immediate obstetrical concerns may prompt emergent delivery peri-cannulation; obstetric and neonatal teams should be on hand. If not already at a center with the capability for multidisciplinary ECMO and MFM care, consultation with such a center to assess ECMO candidacy and potential transfer should be considered, especially for those who have not yet reached 32 weeks gestation and should not pursue controlled delivery.

SUMMARY

Recommendations for the optimal care of pregnant patients with COVID-19 infection are mostly extrapolated from study data involving nonpregnant patients, animals, and separate disease states. In general, the management of pregnant patients for both targeted COVID-19 therapies as well as general critical illness mirrors that of nonpregnant patients, and the therapeutic options for each level of illness severity should not be withheld due to gravid state. Ultimately, vaccination is the mainstay of prevention of poor COVID-19 outcomes, and tailoring COVID-19 disease management for pregnant patients will require research to address the many areas of limited evidence.

CLINICS CARE POINTS

- Appropriate COVID therapies should not be withheld solely due to a pregnant state. Up-to-date COVID therapeutic guidlines can be found online on the NIH website: www. covid19treatmentguidelines.nih.gov/.

- For patients requiring hospitalization in their third trimester of pregnancy, transfer to a facility with maternal-fetal medicine and appropriate neonatal intensive care capability should be considered.

- Stabilization of maternal oxygenation and hemodynamics is the best way to stabilize fetal status. While there are no strict criteria to guide timing of intubation, intubation in a controlled setting with the most capable provider is likely to yield the best outcomes.

REFERENCES

1. Overton EE, Goffman D, Friedman AM. The Epidemiology of COVID-19 in Pregnancy. Clin Obstet Gynecol 2022;65(1):110–22.
2. Schell RC, Macias DA, Garner WH, et al. Examining the impact of trimester of diagnosis on COVID-19 disease progression in pregnancy. Am J Obstet Gynecol MFM 2022;4(6):100728.
3. Zambrano LD, Ellington S, Strid P, et al. CDC COVID-19 Response Pregnancy and Infant Linked Outcomes Team. Update: Characteristics of Symptomatic Women of Reproductive Age with Laboratory-Confirmed SARS-CoV-2 Infection by Pregnancy Status – United States, January 22-October 3, 2020. US Dept of HHS/CDC MMWR 2020;69(44):1641–7.
4. Khan DSA, Pirzada AN, Ali A, et al. The differences in clinical presentation, management, and prognosis of laboratory-confirmed COVID-19 between Pregnant and Non-Pregnant Women: a systematic review and meta-analysis. Int J Environ Res Public Health 2021;18:5613.

5. Halscott T, Vaught J, SMFM COVID-19 Task Force. Society for Maternal-Fetal Medicine Management Considerations for Pregnant Patients With COVID-19. Society for Maternal-Fetal Medicine. Available at: https://www.smfm.org/covidclinical. Accessed 21 Nov 2022.

6. American College of Obstetricians and Gynecologists. COVID-19 FAQs for obstetricians-gynecologists, obstetrics. Washington, DC: ACOG. 2020. Available at: https://www.acog.org/clinical-information/physician-faqs/covid-19-faqs-for-ob-gyns-obstetrics. Accessed 15 Oct 2022.

7. National Institutes of Health COVID-19 Treatment Guidelines Panel. Special Considerations in Pregnancy. 2022. Available at: https://www.covid19treatmentguidelines.nih.gov/special-populations/pregnancy/. Accessed 21 Nov 2022.

8. Therapeutics and COVID-19: living guideline, 22 april 2022. Geneva: World Health Organization; 2022. WHO/2019-nCoV/therapeutics/2022.3). Licence: CC BY-NC-SA 3.0 IGO.

9. Tremblay E, Thérasse E, Thomassin-Naggara I, et al. Quality initiatives: guidelines for use of medical imaging during pregnancy and lactation. Radiographics 2012; 32(3):897–911.

10. National Institutes of Health COVID-19 Treatment Guidelines Panel. Clinical management of adults. 2022. Available at: https://www.covid19treatmentguidelines.nih.gov/management/clinical-management-of-adults/. Accessed 22 Nov 2022.

11. Hammond J, Leister-Tebbe H, Gardner A, et al. Oral Nirmatrelvir for High-Risk, Nonhospitalized Adults with Covid-19. N Engl J Med 2022;386(15):1397–408.

12. Catlin NR, Bowman CJ, Campion SN, et al. Reproductive and developmental safety of nirmatrelvir (PF-07321332), an oral SARS-CoV-2 M^{pro} inhibitor in animal models. Reprod Toxicol 2022;108:56–61.

13. Loza A, Farias R, Gavin N, et al. Short-term pregnancy outcomes after nirmatrelvir-ritonavir treatment for mild-to-moderate coronavirus disease 2019 (COVID-19). Obstet Gynecol 2022;140(3):447–9.

14. Beigel JH, Tomashek KM, Dodd LE, et al. for the ACTT-1 Study Group Members. remdesivir for the Treatment of Covid-19 – Final Report. N Engl J Med 2020;383: 1813–26.

15. Gottlieb RL, Vaca CE, Paredes R, et al. for the PINETREE Investigators. Early Remdesivir to Prevent Progression to Severe Covid-19 in Outpatients. N Engl J Med 2022;386:305–15.

16. Eid J, Abdelwahab M, Colburn N, et al. Early Administration of Remdesivir and Intensive Care Unit Admission in Hospitalized Pregnant Individuals With Coronavirus Disease 2019 (COVID-19). Obstet Gynecol 2022;139(4):619–21.

17. Saroyo YB, Rumondang A, Febriana IS, et al. Remdesivir Treatment for COVID 19 in Pregnant Patients with Moderate to Severe Symptoms: Serial Case Report. Infect Dis Rep 2021;13:437–43.

18. Budi DS, Pratama NR, Wafa IA, et al. Remdesivir for pregnancy: a systematic review of antiviral therapy for COVID-19. Heliyon 2022;8(1):e08835.

19. Singh AK, Singh A, Singh R, et al. Remdesivir in COVID-19: a critical review of pharmacology, pre-clinical and clinical studies. Diabetes Metab Syndr 2020; 14(4):641–8.

20. Mulangu S, Dodd LE, Davey RT Jr. A randomized, controlled trial of Ebola virus disease therapeutics. N Engl J Med 2019;381:2293–303.

21. Waters MD, Warren S, Hughes C, et al. Human genetic risk of treatment with antiviral nucleoside analog drugs that induce lethal mutagenesis: The special case of molnupiravir. Environ Mol Mutagen 2022;63(1):37–63.

22. Montgomery H, Hobbs FDR, Padilla F, et al. TACKLE study group. Efficacy and safety of intramuscular administration of tixagevimab-cilgavimab for early outpatient treatment of COVID-19 (TACKLE): a phase 3, randomised, double-blind, placebo-controlled trial. Lancet Respir Med 2022;10(10):985–96.

23. Ginde AA, Paredes R, Murray TA, et al. ACTIV-3–Therapeutics for Inpatients with COVID-19 (TICO) Study Group. Tixagevimab-cilgavimab for treatment of patients hospitalised with COVID-19: a randomised, double-blind, phase 3 trial. Lancet Respir Med 2022;10(10):972–84.

24. U.S. Food and Drug Administration. Coronavirus (COVID-19) Drugs. 2022. Available at: https://www.fda.gov/drugs/emergency-preparedness-drugs/coronavirus-covid-19-drugs. Accessed 21 Nov 2022.

25. Hirshberg JS, Cooke E, Oakes MC, et al. Monoclonal antibody treatment of symptomatic COVID-19 in pregnancy: initial report. Am J Obstet Gynecol 2021;225(6):688–9.

26. Mayer C, VanHise K, Caskey R, et al. Monoclonal Antibodies Casirivimab and Imdevimab in Pregnancy for Coronavirus Disease 2019 (COVID-19). Obstet Gynecol 2021;138(6):937–9.

27. Thilagar BP, Ghosh AK, Nguyen J, et al. Anti-spike monoclonal antibody therapy in pregnant women with mild-to-moderate coronavirus disease 2019 (COVID-19). Obstet Gynecol 2022;139(4):616–8.

28. Chang MH, Cowman K, Guo Y, et al. A real-world assessment of tolerability and treatment outcomes of COVID-19 monoclonal antibodies administered in pregnancy. Am J Obstet Gynecol 2022;226(5):743–5.

29. Richley M, Rao RR, Afshar Y, et al. Neutralizing monoclonal antibodies for coronavirus disease 2019 (COVID-19) in pregnancy: a case series. Obstet Gynecol 2022;139(3):368–72.

30. Buonomo AR, Esposito N, Di Filippo I, et al. Safety and efficacy of anti-SARS-CoV-2 monoclonal antibodies in pregnancy. Expert Opin Drug Saf 2022 Sep;21(9):1137–41.

31. Bhimraj A, Morgan RL, Shumaker AH, et al. Infectious diseases society of America guidelines on the treatment and management of patients with COVID-19. Infectious Diseases Society of America. 2022. Version 10.1.1. Available at: https://www.idsociety.org/practice-guideline/covid-19-guideline-treatment-and-management/. Accessed 22 Nov 2022.

32. Marconi VC, Ramanan AV, de Bono S, et al. on behalf of the COV-BARRIER Study Group. Efficacy and safety of baricitinib for the treatment of hospitalised adults with COVID-19 (COV-BARRIER): a randomised, double-blind, parallel-group, placebo- controlled phase 3 trial. Lancet Respir Med 2021;9:1407–18.

33. Kalil AC, Patterson TF, Mehta AK, et al. for the ACTT-2 Study Group Members. Baricitinib plus Remdesivir for Hospitalized Adults with Covid-19. N Engl J Med 2021;384:795–807.

34. Guimaraes PO, Quirk D, Furtado RH, et al. for the STOP-COVID Trial Investigators. Tofacitinib in Patients Hospitalized with Covid-19 Pneumonia. N Engl J Med 2021;385:406–15.

35. Gouverneur A, Avouac J, Prati C, et al. JAK inhibitors and risk of major cardiovascular events or venous thromboembolism: a self-controlled case series study. Eur J Clin Pharmacol 2022;78(12):1981–90.

36. Mahadevan U, Dubinsky MC, Su C, et al. Outcomes of Pregnancies With Maternal/Paternal Exposure in the Tofacitinib Safety Databases for Ulcerative Colitis. Inflamm Bowel Dis 2018;24(12):2494–500.

37. Clowse ME, Feldman SR, Isaacs JD, et al. Pregnancy Outcomes in the Tofacitinib Safety Databases for Rheumatoid Arthritis and Psoriasis. Drug Saf 2016;39(8): 755–62.
38. Costanzo G, Firinu D, Losa F, et al. Baricitinib exposure during pregnancy in rheumatoid arthritis. Ther Adv Musculoskelet Dis 2020;12. 1759720X19899296.
39. RECOVERY Collaborative Group. Tocilizumab in patients admitted to hospital with COVID-19 (RECOVERY): a randomised, controlled, open-label, platform trial. Lancet 2021;397:1637–45.
40. Gordon AC, Mouncey PR, Al-Beidh F, et al. The REMAP-CAP Investigators. Interleukin-6 Receptor Antagonists in Critically Ill Patients with Covid-19. N Engl J Med 2021;384:1491–502.
41. Nakajima K, Watanabe O, Mochizuki M, et al. Pregnancy outcomes after exposure to tocilizumab: a retrospective analysis of 61 patients in Japan. Mod Rheumatol 2016;26(5):667–71.
42. Hoeltzenbein M, Beck E, Rajwanshi R, et al. Tocilizumab use in pregnancy: analysis of a global safety database including data from clinical trials and post-marketing data. Semin Arthritis Rheum 2016;46(2):238–45.
43. Jimenez-Lozano I, Caro-Teller JM, Fernandez-Hidalgo N, et al. Safety of tocilizumab in COVID-19 pregnant women and their newborn: A retrospective study. J Clin Pharm Ther 2021;46:1062–70.
44. Jorgensen SCJ, Lapinsky SE. Tocilizumab for coronavirus disease 2019 in pregnancy and lactation: a narrative review. Clin Microbiol Infect 2022;28:51–5.
45. Abdullah S, Bashir N, Mahmood N. Use of intravenous tocilizumab in pregnancy for severe coronavirus disease 2019 pneumonia: two case reports. J Med Case Rep 2021;15:426.
46. The RECOVERY Collaborative Group. Dexamethasone in Hospitalized Patients with Covid-19. N Engl J Med 2021;384:693–704.
47. Villar J, Ferrando C, Martínez D, et al. Dexamethasone treatment for the acute respiratory distress syndrome: a multicentre, randomised controlled trial. Lancet Respir Med 2020;e(3):267–76.
48. Tomazini BM, Maia IS, Cavalcanti AB, et al. for the COALITION COVID-19 Brazil III Investigators. Effect of Dexamethasone on Days Alive and Ventilator-Free in Patients With Moderate or Severe Acute Respiratory Distress Syndrome and COVID-19: The CoDEX Randomized Clinical Trial. JAMA 2020;324(13):1307–16.
49. Sterne JAC, Murthy S, Diaz JV, REACT Working Group. Association Between Administration of Systemic Corticosteroids and Mortality Among Critically Ill Patients With COVID-19: A Meta-analysis. JAMA 2020;324(13):1330–41.
50. Granholm A, Munch MW, Myatra SN, et al. Dexamethasone 12 mg versus 6 mg for patients with COVID-19 and severe hypoxaemia: a pre-planned, secondary Bayesian analysis of the COVID STEROID 2 trial. Intensive Care Med 2022;48(1):45–55.
51. Hu KM, Hong AS. Resuscitating the crashing pregnant patient. Emerg Med Clin North Am 2020;38(4):903–17.
52. Wang C, Xu YJ, Shi Y, et al. Verification on the developmental toxicity of short-term exposure to phenol in rats. Biomed Environ Sci 2020;33(6):403–13.
53. Guerin C, Reignier J, Richard J-C, et al, for the PROSEVA Study Group. Prone Positioning in Severe Acute Respiratory Distress Syndrome. N Engl J Med 2013;368:2159–68.
54. Thompson AE, Ranard BL, Wei Y, et al. Prone Positioning in Awake, Nonintubated Patients With COVID-19 Hypoxemic Respiratory Failure. JAMA Intern Med 2020; 180(11):1537–9.

55. Ehrmann S, Li J, Ibarra-Estrata M, et al. for the Awake Prone Positioning Meta-Trial Group. Awake prone positioning for COVID-19 acute hypoxaemic respiratory failure: a randomised, controlled, multinational, open-label meta-trial. Lancet Respir Med 2021;9:1387–95.
56. Pourdowlat G, Mikaeilvand A, Eftekhariyazdi M, et al. Prone-Position Ventilation in a Pregnant Woman with Severe COVID-19 Infection Associated with Acute Respiratory Distress Syndrome. Tanaffos 2020;19(2):152–5.
57. Alhazzani W, Parhar KKS, Weatherald J, et al. Effect of Awake Prone Positioning on Endotracheal Intubation in Patients With COVID-19 and Acute Respiratory Failure: A Randomized Clinical Trial. JAMA 2022;327(21):2104–13.
58. Ni Y-N, Luo J, Yu H, et al. The effect of high-flow nasal cannula in reducing the mortality and the rate of endotracheal intubation when used before mechanical ventilation compared with conventional oxygen therapy and noninvasive positive pressure ventilation. A systematic review and meta-analysis. Am J Emerg Med 2018;36:226–33.
59. Riera J, Barbeta E, Tormos A, et al. CIBERESUCICOVID Consortium. Effects of intubation timing in patients with COVID-19 throughout the four waves of the pandemic: a matched analysis. Eur Respir J 2023 Mar 2;63(3):2201426. https://doi.org/10.1183/13993003.01426-2022. PMID: 36396142; PMCID: PMC9686319.
60. Kang BJ, Koh Y, Lim CM, et al. Failure of high-flow nasal cannula therapy may delay intubation and increase mortality. Intensive Care Med 2015;41(4):623–32.
61. Nishikimi M, Nishida K, Shindo Y, et al. Failure of non-invasive respiratory support after 6 hours from initiation is associated with ICU mortality. PLoS One 2021;16(4): e0251030.
62. Oxford-Horrey C, Savage M, Prabhu M, et al. Putting It All Together: Clinical Considerations in the Care of Critically Ill Obstetric Patients with COVID-19. Am J Perinatol 2020;37(10):1044–51.
63. Chanques G, Constantin JM, Devlin JW, et al. Analgesia and sedation in patients with ARDS. Intensive Care Med 2020;46(12):2342–56.
64. Stephens RJ, Evans EM, Pajor MJ, et al. A dual-center cohort study on the association between early deep sedation and clinical outcomes in mechanically ventilated patients during the COVID-19 pandemic: The COVID-SED study. Crit Care 2022;26(1):179.
65. Stephens RJ, Ablordeppey E, Drewry AM, et al. Analgosedation Practices and the Impact of Sedation Depth on Clinical Outcomes Among Patients Requiring Mechanical Ventilation in the ED: A Cohort Study. Chest 2017;152(5):963–71.
66. Wiedemann HP, Wheeler AP, Bernard GR, et al. Comparison of two fluid-management strategies in acute lung injury. N Engl J Med 2006;354(24):2564–75.
67. Manuck TA, Rice MM, Bailit JL, et al. Eunice Kennedy Shriver National Institute of Child Health and Human Development Maternal-Fetal Medicine Units Network. Preterm neonatal morbidity and mortality by gestational age: a contemporary cohort. Am J Obstet Gynecol 2016;215(1):103.e1–14.
68. Chong J, Ahmed S, Hill K. Acute respiratory distress syndrome in a pregnant patient with COVID-19 improved after delivery: a case report and brief review. Respir Med Case Rep 2020;31:101171.
69. Pineles BL, Stephens A, Narendran LM, et al. Does delivery affect time to recovery in COVID-19-related ARDS during pregnancy? Am J Obstet Gynecol 2021; 224(2):S498–9.

Resuscitation of the Obstetric Patient

Cheyenne Snavely, MD[a,*], Caleb Chan, MD[a,b]

KEYWORDS

- Resuscitation • Critical care • Obstetrics • Pregnancy • Emergency medicine

KEY POINTS

- During acute resuscitation, neither necessary medications nor diagnostic imaging should be withheld from a pregnant woman because of fetal concerns.
- Call consultants and prepare obstetric and neonatal-specific equipment early when caring for a critically ill pregnant patient.
- Anticipate anatomically difficult and physiologically tenuous intubation in the obstetric patient.
- Target a PaO_2 > 70 mm Hg, $PaCO_2$ of 30 to 60 mm Hg, and maternal pH 7.25 to 7.35 in obstetric patients with acute respiratory distress syndrome.
- Patients in later stages of pregnancy with hemodynamic instability or cardiac arrest should be placed in a supine position with the uterus manually displaced toward the patient's left.
- Perimortem cesarean section should be performed within 5 minutes from the time of the cardiac arrest.

INTRODUCTION
Epidemiology

In 2018, there were 143.5 million emergency department visits.[1] Of these, 5.9% received a diagnosis of pregnancy, childbirth, or puerperium-related illness, and 3.1% required hospital admission.[1] Maternal mortality in the United States is on the rise, from 658 in 2018 to 754 in 2019, and 861 in 2020.[2] It is notable that there are significant racial and ethnic disparities related to maternal mortality with non-Hispanic Black women being at the highest risk followed by non-Hispanic American Indian or Alaska Native women.[3] Maternal mortality is defined by the World Health Organization (WHO) as "the annual number of female deaths from any cause related to or aggravated by pregnancy or its management (excluding accidental or incidental causes)

[a] Department of Medicine, University of Maryland Medical Center, 110 South Paca Street, 6th Floor, Suite 200, Baltimore, MD 21201, USA; [b] Department of Emergency Medicine, University of Maryland School of Medicine, 110 South Paca Street, 6th Floor, Suite 200, Baltimore, MD 21201, USA
* Corresponding author. 110 South Paca Street, 6th Floor, Suite 200, Baltimore, MD 21201.
E-mail address: chey.snav@gmail.com

Emerg Med Clin N Am 41 (2023) 323–335
https://doi.org/10.1016/j.emc.2022.12.005
0733-8627/23/© 2022 Elsevier Inc. All rights reserved.
emed.theclinics.com

during childbirth or within 42 days of termination of pregnancy."[4] The most common cause of pregnancy-related mortality in the United States are cardiovascular conditions (**Table 1**).[3] Maternal mortality due to traumatic injury is not reported in the standard pregnancy-related mortality statistics used by the Center for Disease Control or WHO, and therefore the impact of trauma in pregnancy is often underappreciated. Traumatic injury during pregnancy is the leading cause of non-obstetric maternal mortality accounting for ~20% of maternal deaths.[5] The most common cause of trauma in pregnancy is motor vehicle collision (58%) followed by falls (17%) and assaults (15%).[6] A recent meta-analysis demonstrated a 9% prevalence of physical intimate partner violence in pregnancy in North America.[7]

Physiologic Changes of Pregnancy

To aid with diagnosis and management, emergency medicine physicians must understand the normal physiologic changes that occur during pregnancy (**Table 2**).[8] The driver of these changes are increased metabolic demand and diversion of blood flow to the fetus. These physiologic changes serve to support the fetus and mother during pregnancy, however, they come at a cost of decreasing physiologic reserves which normally would be called upon during critical illness. Understanding these areas of susceptibility is crucial to managing a crashing obstetric patient.

DISCUSSION
Airway Management in the Obstetric Patient

For all-comers to the ED, the first-pass success rate for intubations is ~83%, with an overall success rate of 99.4%.[9] The incidence of failed intubations in pregnant patients is estimated to be eight times higher than for non-pregnant patients.[10] Factors that likely contribute to a more difficult airway include but are not limited to laryngeal edema, increased vascularity of airways, decreased buffering capacity for elevations in carbon dioxide, and rapid oxygen desaturation.[8]

These changes reinforce the importance of first-pass success in the pregnant patient and the significance of maximizing optimization before intubation.[11] Important factors include pre-oxygenation and apneic oxygenation, selecting the appropriate

Table 1 Causes of pregnancy-related deaths in the United States from 2014 to 2017[3]	
Etiology	**Percentage**
Other cardiovascular conditions	15.5%
Infection or sepsis	12.7%
Other noncardiovascular medical conditions	12.5%
Cardiomyopathy	11.5%
Hemorrhage	10.7%
Thrombotic pulmonary or other embolisms	9.6%
Cerebrovascular accidents	8.2%
Unknown	6.7%
Hypertensive disorders of pregnancy	6.6%
Amniotic fluid embolism	5.5%
Anesthesia complications	0.4%

Data from [Reproductive Health: Pregnancy Mortality Surveillance System. Centers for Disease Control and Prevention. Published April 13, 2022. Accessed June 5, 2022] (**Table 1**).

Table 2
Physiologic changes associated with pregnancy[8]

System	Changes	Consequence
Cardiovascular	*Increased*	Higher CPR demands
	Heart rate (15 to 20 bpm)	Increased risk of
	Cardiac output (~40%)	supraventricular tachycardia
	Plasma volume	Third spacing of fluids
	Dilutional anemia	
	Estrogen	
	Decreased	
	Supine blood pressure	
	Systemic vascular resistance	
	Oncotic pressure	
Respiratory/pulmonary	*Increased*	Decreased buffering capacity
	Minute ventilation	Rapid hypoxia
	Oxygen consumption	Difficult intubation
	Laryngeal edema	Decreased ventilation capacity
	Decreased	Increased compression force
	Functional residual capacity	
	$PaCO_2$	
	Chest wall compliance	
Renal/GU	Decreased serum bicarb	Decreased buffering capacity and increased acidemia during CPR
Gastrointestinal	Decreased gastroesophageal sphincter tone	Increased risk of aspiration
Uteroplacental	*Increased*	Sequesters blood in CPR
	Blood flow (~30% of cardiac output)	Contributes to hemodynamic instability
	Aortocaval compression	Requires chest tube placement
	Elevation of diaphragm	higher than for non-pregnant patients
Hematology	Increased clotting factors	Increased risk of venous thromboembolism

Data from [ACOG Practice Bulletin No. 211: Critical Care in Pregnancy. Obstet Gynecol. 2019;133(5):e303-e319. doi:10.1097/AOG.0000000000003241].

equipment, and choosing the most experienced operator.[12] For pregnant patients, it is recommended that a smaller endotracheal tube be used given the high prevalence of laryngeal edema.[12] There are mixed data regarding the use of direct versus video laryngoscopy (DL vs VL) in the general population; however, there are no specific data regarding its use in the obstetric population. For inexperienced operators, VL is likely to have a higher first-pass success rate, however, this is not always true for experienced operators.[13] Ultimately, the difficult airway literature suggests that first-pass success is higher with VL and therefore this is often recommended for use in the pregnant airway.[14]

Pregnant patients also have a higher risk of aspiration due to decreased gastro-esophageal sphincter tone, which can contribute to morbidity and mortality. Rapid sequence intubation and intubation with the head of the bed elevated to 20 to 30° is recommended to mitigate these risks.[12,15]

Studies show that neuromuscular blockade increases the first-pass success rate and decreases procedure-related complications.[16,17] Although anesthesia literature suggests that the first-pass success rate is higher with succinylcholine as compared with rocuronium, other studies have found that first-pass success rate or peri-intubation complications are not affected by the agent chosen for neuromuscular blockade.[18,19] Some argue that succinylcholine at 1.5 mg/kg is the medication of choice for obstetric airways because of its shorter duration of action which allows for a quicker return of spontaneous breathing in case of a difficult airway.[20] However, other studies argue that the time to critical desaturation, defined as SpO2 <80%, was met before the return of significant neuromuscular function for succinylcholine, which may be related to the increase in oxygenation consumption associated with the use of succinylcholine.[21,22] Moreover, if multiple attempts are required, the neuromuscular blockade from succinylcholine may no longer be in effect.[20] Because obstetric airways are often difficult and may require multiple attempts, some advocate for the use of rocuronium at 1.2 mg/kg, especially in settings where sugammadex is available.[20] It should be noted that prior data suggest the reversal of rocuronium is 2.9 min faster than spontaneous recovery from succinylcholine.[23] Although the time of onset does not differ significantly for neuromuscular blockade in pregnancy, the duration of action can be longer for women in their second and third trimesters.[24] When used in appropriate doses, neither depolarizing nor nondepolarizing agents should cross the placenta.[25]

For induction agents, hemodynamic effects are often the dominating factors that guide decision-making. In 2013, thiopental was the most common induction agent used for obstetric patients undergoing general anesthesia in the United Kingdom.[26] In the United States, thiopental has fallen out of favor due to its concern for hemodynamic compromise and lack of availability.[27–29] Instead, propofol is often preferred and has added benefits because it does not decrease uterine muscle tone.[12] Although not specific to obstetric patients, a recent study of patients in the intensive care unit demonstrated more favorable outcomes with the use of propofol over ketamine or etomidate for induction in rapid sequence intubation.[30] That being said, etomidate is often the agent of choice for emergency room physicians.[31,32]

Breathing and Mechanical Ventilation in the Obstetric Patient

Factors that affect breathing and mechanical ventilation in pregnant patients include an elevated diaphragm, a decreased functional residual capacity, decreased chest wall compliance, increased oxygen consumption, and carbon dioxide production, in the setting of chronic respiratory alkalosis with metabolic compensation.[8,33]

It is important to note that although pregnant patients were excluded from the practice-changing ARDSnet trial, the same principles are often broadly applied to this population. Similar to the standard of care for non-pregnant patients, low tidal volume ventilation is recommended for mechanically ventilated pregnant patients.[34]

There is some literature to support modifications to standard mechanical ventilation strategies for obstetric patients. Although a target SpO2 > 88% (PaO2 > 55 mm Hg) is reasonable in most patients with acute respiratory distress syndrome, in pregnant patients the target should be an SpO2 > 95% or a PaO2 >70 mm Hg. The reason for this higher target is that oxygen delivery to the fetus is determined largely by maternal arterial oxygen content. Other important factors are uterine blood flow, concentration of hemoglobin, and the hemoglobin oxygen dissociation curve.[33,35] Maternal hypoxia results in fetoplacental vasoconstriction thereby limiting blood flow and oxygen delivery.[36] This can also occur due to catecholamines, alkalosis, hypotension, and contractions.[36] Uteroplacental oxygen delivery can often be improved by increasing cardiac output, blood transfusions, and by optimizing the mother's oxygenation.[37] In addition, PaCO2 should not be below 30 or above 60 mm Hg, with maternal pH 7.25 to 7.35 (compared with 7.3 to 7.45 in the general population).[33,38] Patients in their third trimester generally have decreased pulmonary compliance and may benefit from higher PEEP, though caution is advised given the consequential reduction in cardiac preload and potentially cardiac output.[33–35] Pregnant women can be placed in prone positioning with appropriate padding, but lateral positioning may be more feasible.[35]

A wider differential for respiratory failure should be considered in the pregnant population. Some obstetric-specific causes of acute respiratory failure include preeclampsia, amniotic fluid embolism, and side effects of tocolytic administration.[39] *Amniotic fluid embolism* is a rare but often fatal complication that occurs during labor, cesarean delivery, dilation and evacuation, or within 30 min of the postpartum period. It presents with acute hypoxia, hypotension, coagulopathy or hemorrhage, and can progress to cardiac arrest. Treatment is supportive in addition to delivery of the fetus if this has not occurred already.[40]

Circulatory Support in the Obstetric Patient with Shock

Shock due to trauma

The primary survey for the obstetric trauma patient is unchanged; however, it should include the addition of manual left uterine displacement.[41] In addition, if a deep peritoneal lavage is required, it is recommended to use an open technique after bladder and stomach decompression.[42]

The focused assessment sonography in trauma (FAST) can and should be completed, and has similar sensitivities to the non-pregnant population.[41] If further imaging is necessary, it should never be withheld out of concern for fetal harm.

A vaginal exam should be done as a part of the secondary evaluation, but it should be noted that an ultrasound must first rule out placenta previa in patients greater than 23 weeks gestational age (GA) with vaginal bleeding.[5]

Continuous fetal heart monitoring for a minimum of 4 to 6 h should be initiated for any woman at greater than 24 weeks GA who has experienced significant trauma.[43]

To prevent complications with future pregnancies, Rho(D) immune globulin is typically administered to obstetric patients presenting with significant trauma.[44] In general, 300 mcg (one vial) protects against 30 mL of fetal blood and is commonly the dose of choice for vaginal bleeding after 12 weeks GA[44] However, in the setting of significant trauma, the Kleihauer-Betke test should be done to determine the proper dosing of Rho(D) immune globulin (**Table 3** for dosing specifics).[44] In addition to Rho(D) immune globulin, the tetanus toxoid should be administered when indicated.[43]

For a *pneumothorax or hemothorax* requiring the placement of a chest tube, recommended placement is in the 3rd or 4th intercostal space, notably higher than in the general population due to uterine displacement of abdominal contents superiorly.[41]

Shock due to Hemorrhage and Specific Pregnancy-related Complications

Ruptured ectopic pregnancies were the primary cause of hemorrhage-related maternal mortality in the United States from 2011 to 2013.[45] Ruptured ectopic pregnancies can present in many different ways, however, they most commonly present during the first trimester with abdominal pain and vaginal bleeding.[46] Diagnosis is typically made with ultrasound and human chorionic gonadotropin testing. Although medical management can be an option for non-ruptured ectopic pregnancies, the mainstay of treatment for a ruptured ectopic is surgical management in addition to resuscitation.[46]

Placental abruption is a feared complication of trauma and has a reported maternal mortality as high as 53%.[47] It is a result of placental separation from the uterus and can result in either retroplacental or vaginal bleeding.[47] The most common symptoms are tachycardia, low blood pressure, a firm and painful abdomen and signs of fetal

Table 3
Medication considerations and dosing in obstetric emergencies[7,20,44,51,53,54,65,68]

Indication	Treatment Options	Special Considerations
Pre-eclampsia/eclampsia	*Labetalol* 10 to 20 mg IV, then 20 to 80 every 10 to 30 min (max dose 300 mg), or continuous infusion of 1 to 2 mg/min *Hydralazine* 5 mg IV or IM, then 5 to 10 mg IV every 20 to 40 min (max dose 20 mg), or continuous infusion of 0.5 to 10 mg/hr *Magnesium* 4 to 6 mg IV over 20 to 30 min or 10 mg IM followed by 1 to 2 g/hr IV	Caution in patients with asthma, bradycardia, or significant cardiac dysfunction Caution in patients with renal dysfunction
Postpartum hemorrhage	*Oxytocin* 10 to 40 units in 500 to 1000 mL as a continuous infusion or 10 units IM *Misoprostol* 1000 mcg per rectum *Methylergonovine* 0.2 mg IM *Carboprost tromethamine* 0.25 mg IM *Tranexamic acid* 1g IV, can repeat at 30 min if persistent bleeding	Contraindicated in hypertensive patients
Tocolysis	*Terbutaline* 0.25 mg SQ	Should be given in consultation with an obstetrician
Fetomaternal hemorrhage	*RhD immune globulin* For small-volume vaginal bleeding or minor trauma, the standard dose for women at >12 wk GA with minor trauma is 300 mcg For large volume hemorrhage or major trauma: #of vials (300 mcg/vial) = 50/30 x %fetal cells (round to nearest decimal point and then add 1 vial)	Indicated in RhD negative mother's Quantitative Kleihauer-Betke testing determines the % fetal cells in the maternal circulation

distress.[47] Of note, although its specificity is high, ultrasound has poor sensitivity for identifying placental abruption.[47,48] Management includes establishing large bore intravenous (IV) access, potential administration of blood products, and correction of coagulopathy, in addition to fetal monitoring and potential delivery.[49,50]

Placenta previa, a condition where the placenta covers the internal os, can present with painless vaginal bleeding, and in this scenario, it is important to avoid digital vaginal exams.[51] If co-existing contractions occur, tocolysis should be considered with magnesium or terbutaline.[51] The goal of treatment is to stabilize the mother until a cesarean section can be performed and steroids administered if indicated (expected delivery within 7 days and GA between $24^{0/7}$ - $33^{6/7}$) for fetal lung maturity.[51,52]

Postpartum hemorrhage (PPH) is a life-threatening emergency. The most common cause of PPH is uterine atony which can be made worse by drugs like magnesium and nitroglycerin.[51] Management includes uterine massage, tamponade, the administration of blood products, and treatment of coagulopathy if present, additional strategies are outlined in **Fig. 1**.[51]

Tranexamic acid (TXA) has been shown to reduce blood loss and death in the setting of postpartum hemorrhage and should be administered to patients with an estimated blood loss > 500 mL after vaginal delivery or > 1000 mL after cesarean.[53] TXA should be given within 3 hours from time of delivery and can be repeated if bleeding continues at 30 minutes from initial dose or re-occurrence within 24 hours.[53,54]

Uterine rupture is rare but can be catastrophic. Presenting signs may include severe abdominal pain, contractions, vaginal bleeding, fetal distress, signs of hemorrhagic shock and palpable fetal parts on abdominal exam.[55,56] Treatment is stabilization and immediate laparotomy.

Shock due to Vasodilatation and the use of Vasopressors

In theory, ephedrine is thought to elevate blood pressure primarily by increasing cardiac output, with minimal peripheral vasoconstriction thereby minimizing the risk of decreasing uteroplacental blood flow.[57] However, its slow onset of action and difficulty with titration make its use in critical illness challenging.[57] There is minimal data for the use of vasopressors in the septic obstetric patient. Most experts advocate for standard of care based on the Surviving Sepsis guidelines which recommend norepinephrine as the first line and vasopressin as the second line agent.[8,58] Although norepinephrine causes peripheral vasoconstriction, recent animal data suggest it has the least effect on the uterine artery when compared with other commonly used vasoactive drugs such as phenylephrine and vasopressin.[59] Ultimately, no agents should be withheld out of fear for induction of uterine contractions or decreased uteroplacental blood flow.

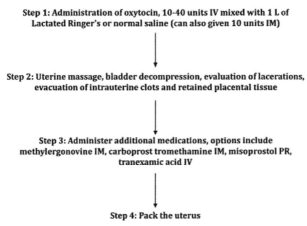

Fig. 1. Proposed strategy for the treatment of the undifferentiated postpartum hemorrhage.[51,53,54] IV, intravenous; IM, intramuscular; PR, per rectum.

Cardiac Arrest

Cardiac arrest in pregnancy is rare, estimated at 1 in 30,000 pregnancies.[60] Acute cardiovascular life support (ACLS) for pregnant and non-pregnant patients suffering from a cardiac arrest is nearly identical with a few exceptions.[61] Manual left uterine displacement should be applied for the duration of cardiopulmonary resuscitation (CPR).[61] The use of mechanical compression devices in pregnancy should be avoided due to a paucity of data.[61] Similar to ACLS for all-comers, continuous waveform capnography can be used to help determine adequacy of chest compressions (adequate >10 mm Hg).[61] Defibrillation pads should be placed in the anterolateral position.[61] Medications should be given through an IV access point above the diaphragm.[61]

Upon notification of a pregnant patient in cardiac arrest, obstetric and neonatal consultants should be immediately called and additional equipment should be requested to be brought to the bedside. This includes an antiseptic solution, a number 10 blade scalpel, a Balfour retractor, a pack of sponges, two Kelly clamps, a needle driver, Russian forceps, sutures and suture scissors, and neonatal resuscitation equipment.[61]

A *perimortem cesarean* section is indicated in pregnant patients with a gravid uterus (fundus above the level of the umbilicus) and suspected GA > 20 weeks who are suffering from a cardiac arrest and have not regained return of spontaneous circulation (ROSC).[61] In general, it is recommended that this be initiated within 5 minutes from time of cardiac arrest.[61] If time allows, bladder decompression is ideal but should not delay the procedure.[62] If available, an antiseptic can be used on the abdominal wall.[61] To perform a perimortem cesarean section, an incision is made from the xiphoid to the pubic symphysis with a number 10 blade scalpel. Next, all layers of the abdominal wall are incised with either blunt scissors or the scalpel. The bladder is then manually retracted and the uterus externalized. A short vertical incision is then made through the uterine wall and extended from the fundus toward the bladder with scissors.[62,63] The fetus is then delivered, and the umbilical cord clamped and cut immediately.[62] After the fetus is delivered, the open uterus and abdomen should be packed to minimize bleeding.[63] If ROSC is achieved, the mother should be briskly attended to by a surgical specialist and given prophylactic antibiotics.[63] Manual left uterine displacement and standard ACLS should be continued throughout the duration of the procedure.[61]

Disability Evaluation and Treatment in the Obstetric Patient

In the United States, preeclampsia/eclampsia affects 3.4% of pregnancies.[64] *Preeclampsia* is defined as new onset of hypertension (>140/90 mm Hg on 2 occasions at least 4 h apart with a previously normal blood pressure) associated with proteinuria after 20 weeks GA. Features of severe preeclampsia include thrombocytopenia, abnormalities in liver function, severe persistent right upper quadrant pain, headache, visual disturbances, renal insufficiency and pulmonary edema. A blood pressure > 160/110 mm Hg is also considered a severe feature.[65] *Eclampsia* is a new onset seizure in a pregnant patient without an alternative etiology. It is most common 48 to 72 h postpartum, and can be preceded by headache, blurry vision, photophobia, and altered mental status.[65] In those who have not yet delivered, the ultimate treatment is delivery, which is typically recommended for patients at greater than 37 weeks GA and variably for patients at less than 37 weeks GA.[65]

Magnesium sulfate is the drug of choice for the prevention and treatment of seizures for patients with preeclampsia/eclampsia. Magnesium sulfate is typically given with a loading dose of 4 to 6 g IV over 20 to 30 min, if IV administration is not feasible, an intramuscular dose of 10 g can be administered.[65] The loading dose is followed by a continuous infusion at 1 to 2 g/hr.[65] Patients should be closely monitored for side effects of magnesium administration. These include loss of deep tendon reflexes around a magnesium level of 9 mg/dL, respiratory depression at a level of 12 mg/dL, and rarely, cardiac arrest at levels of 30 mg/dL. If toxicity develops, the recommended treatment is IV administration of 10 mL of 10% calcium gluconate and furosemide.[65]

If the etiology of seizure is unclear, there should be a low threshold for further workup, as pregnant women are also at increased risk for developing cerebral venous sinus thrombosis and strokes which can present with seizures.[66,67]

SUMMARY

Caring for the crashing pregnant patient presents multiple challenges. To best manage these patients, it is important to understand the physiologic changes that occur during pregnancy. This information will aid in both the diagnosis and treatment of these complex patients. It is important to remember that although pregnant women are subject to illnesses exclusive to the obstetric population, they are also susceptible to the same illnesses as the general population, but may present differently due to their altered physiology. In caring for these patients, it is paramount to remember that there are two patients, both the mom and the fetus. However, in the majority of cases, treating the mother's illness will ultimately benefit the fetus.

CLINICS CARE POINTS

- During acute resuscitation, neither necessary medications nor diagnostic imaging should be withheld from a pregnant woman because of fetal concerns
- Call consultants and prepare obstetric and neonatal-specific equipment early when caring for a critically ill pregnant patient
- Anticipate anatomically difficult and physiologically tenuous intubation in the obstetric patient
- Target a PaO_2 > 70 mm Hg, $PaCO_2$ of 30 to 60 mm Hg, and maternal pH 7.25 to 7.35 in obstetric patients with acute respiratory distress syndrome
- Patients in later stages of pregnancy with hemodynamic instability or cardiac arrest should be placed in a supine position with the uterus manually displaced toward the patient's left
- Perimortem cesarean section should be performed within 5 minutes from time of the cardiac arrest

DISCLOSURE

The Authors have nothing to disclose

REFERENCES

1. Weiss AJ, Jiang HJ. Most Frequent Reasons for Emergency Department Visits, 2018. 2021. Available at: https://www.hcup-us.ahrq.gov/reports/statbriefs/sb286-ED-Frequent-Conditions-2018.pdf.
2. Hoyert DL, National Center for Health Statistics. Maternal mortality rates in the united states, 2020. centers for disease control and prevention. 2022. Available

at: https://www.cdc.gov/nchs/data/hestat/maternal-mortality/2020/maternal-mortality-rates-2020.htm. Accessed June 7, 2022.

3. Reproductive Health. Pregnancy mortality surveillance system. Centers Dis Control Prev 2022. Available at: https://www.cdc.gov/reproductivehealth/maternal-mortality/pregnancy-mortality-surveillance-system.htm. Accessed June 5, 2022.

4. World Health Organization. The global health observatory indicator metadata registry list: maternal deaths. Available at: https://www.who.int/data/gho/indicator-metadata-registry/imr-details/4622. Accessed June 7, 2022.

5. Jain V, Chari R, Maslovitz S, et al. Guidelines for the Management of a Pregnant Trauma Patient. J Obstet Gynaecol Can 2015;37(6):553–71.

6. Wilkerson R, Yuan S, Windsor T. Trauma in Pregnancy: A Comprehensive Overview. Relias Media. 2020. Available at: https://www.reliasmedia.com/articles/146057-trauma-in-pregnancy-a-comprehensive-overview. Accessed June 7, 2022.

7. Román-Gálvez RM, Martín-Peláez S, Fernández-Félix BM, et al. Worldwide Prevalence of Intimate Partner Violence in Pregnancy. A Systematic Review and Meta-Analysis. Front Public Health 2021;9. Available at: https://www.frontiersin.org/article/10.3389/fpubh.2021.738459. Accessed March 18, 2022.

8. ACOG Practice Bulletin No. 211. Critical Care in Pregnancy. Obstet Gynecol 2019;133(5):e303–19.

9. Brown CA, Bair AE, Pallin DJ, et al. of Emergency Department Adult Intubations. Ann Emerg Med 2015;65(4):363–70, e1.

10. Quinn AC, Milne D, Columb M, et al. Failed tracheal intubation in obstetric anaesthesia: 2 yr national case–control study in the UK. Br J Anaesth 2013;110(1):74–80.

11. Sakles JC, Chiu S, Mosier J, et al. The Importance of First Pass Success When Performing Orotracheal Intubation in the Emergency Department. Acad Emerg Med 2013;20(1):71–8.

12. Mushambi MC, Kinsella SM, Popat M, et al. Obstetric Anaesthetists' Association and Difficult Airway Society guidelines for the management of difficult and failed tracheal intubation in obstetrics. Anaesthesia 2015;70(11):1286–306.

13. Griesdale DEG, Liu D, McKinney J, et al. Glidescope® video-laryngoscopy versus direct laryngoscopy for endotracheal intubation: a systematic review and meta-analysis. Can J Anesth Can Anesth 2012;59(1):41–52.

14. Scott-Brown S, Russell R. Video laryngoscopes and the obstetric airway. Int J Obstet Anesth 2015;24(2):137–46.

15. Vasdev GM, Harrison BA, Keegan MT, et al. Management of the difficult and failed airway in obstetric anesthesia. J Anesth 2008;22(1):38–48.

16. Mosier JM, Sakles JC, Stolz U, et al. Neuromuscular Blockade Improves First-Attempt Success for Intubation in the Intensive Care Unit. A Propensity Matched Analysis. Ann Am Thorac Soc 2015;12(5):734–41.

17. Wilcox SR, Bittner EA, Elmer J, et al. Neuromuscul. Blocking Agent Administration Emergent Tracheal Intubation Is Associated Decreased Prevalence Procedure-related Complications*. Crit Care Med 2012;40(6):1808–13.

18. April MD, Arana A, Pallin DJ, et al. Emergency Department Intubation Success With Succinylcholine Versus Rocuronium: A National Emergency Airway Registry Study. Ann Emerg Med 2018;72(6):645–53.

19. Tran DT, Newton EK, Mount VA, et al. Rocuronium versus succinylcholine for rapid sequence induction intubation. Cochrane Database Syst Rev 2015;2015(10):CD002788.

20. Chaggar R, Campbell J. The future of general anaesthesia in obstetrics. BJA Educ 2017;17(3):79–83.
21. Benumof JL, Dagg R, Benumof R. Critical Hemoglobin Desaturation Will Occur before Return to an Unparalyzed State following 1 mg/kg Intravenous Succinylcholine. Anesthesiology 1997;87:979–82.
22. Taha SK, El-Khatib MF, Baraka AS, et al. Effect of suxamethonium vs rocuronium on onset of oxygen desaturation during apnoea following rapid sequence induction. Anaesthesia 2010;65(4):358–61.
23. Lee C, Jahr JS, Candiotti KA, et al. Reversal of Profound Neuromuscular Block by Sugammadex Administered Three Minutes after Rocuronium. Anesthesiology 2009;110(5):1020–5.
24. Jun IJ, Jun J, Kim EM, et al. Comparison of rocuronium-induced neuromuscular blockade in second trimester pregnant women and non-pregnant women. Int J Obstet Anesth 2018;34:10–4.
25. Shin J. Anesthetic Management of the Pregnant Patient: Part 2. Anesth Prog 2021;68(2):119–27.
26. Murdoch H, Scrutton M, Laxton CH. Choice of anaesthetic agents for caesarean section: A UK survey of current practice. Int J Obstet Anesth 2013;22(1):31–5.
27. Sivilotti ML, Ducharme J. Randomized, Double-Blind Study on Sedatives and Hemodynamics During Rapid-Sequence Intubation in the Emergency Department: The SHRED Study. Ann Emerg Med 1998;31(3):313–24.
28. Rucklidge M. Up-to-date or out-of-date: does thiopental have a future in obstetric general anaesthesia? Int J Obstet Anesth 2013;22(3):175–8.
29. Devroe S, Van de Velde M, Rex S. General anesthesia for caesarean section. Curr Opin Anesthesiol 2015;28(3):240–6.
30. Wan C, Hanson AC, Schulte PJ, et al. Propofol, Ketamine, and Etomidate as Induction Agents for Intubation and Outcomes in Critically Ill Patients: A Retrospective Cohort Study. Crit Care Explor 2021;3(5):e0435.
31. Bergen JM, Smith DC. A review of etomidate for rapid sequence intubation in the emergency department. J Emerg Med 1997;15(2):221–30.
32. Sharda SC, Bhatia MS. Etomidate Compared with Ketamine for Induction during Rapid Sequence Intubation: A Systematic Review and Meta-analysis. Indian J Crit Care Med Peer-rev Off Publ Indian Soc Crit Care Med 2022;26(1):108–13.
33. Schwaiberger D, Karcz M, Menk M, et al. Ventilation in the Pregnant Patient. Crit Care Clin 2016;32(1):85–95.
34. Gutiérrez MAG. Considerations for Mechanical Ventilation in the Critically Ill Obstetric Patient. Crit Care Obstet Gynecol 2020;8. https://doi.org/10.36648/2471-9803.6.4.10.
35. Troiano NH, Richter A, King C. Acute Respiratory Failure and Mechanical Ventilation in Women With COVID-19 During Pregnancy: Best Clinical Practices. J Perinat Neonatal Nurs 2022;36(1):27–36.
36. Hampl V, Jakoubek V. Regulation of fetoplacental vascular bed by hypoxia. Physiol Res 2009;58(Suppl 2):S87–94.
37. Lapinsky SE. Cardiopulmonary Complications Pregnancy: Crit Care Med 2005;33(7):1616–22.
38. NHLBI ARDS Network | Tools. Available at: http://www.ardsnet.org/tools.shtml. Accessed June 6, 2022.
39. Bhatia PK, Biyani G, Mohammed S, et al. Acute respiratory failure and mechanical ventilation in pregnant patient: A narrative review of literature. J Anaesthesiol Clin Pharmacol 2016;32(4):431–9.

40. Kaur K, Bhardwaj M, Kumar P, et al. Amniotic fluid embolism. J Anaesthesiol Clin Pharmacol 2016;32(2):153–9.
41. Mendez-Figueroa H, Dahlke JD, Vrees RA, et al. Trauma in pregnancy: an updated systematic review. Am J Obstet Gynecol 2013;209(1):1–10.
42. Nagy KK, Roberts RR, Joseph KT, et al. Experience with over 2500 diagnostic peritoneal lavages. Injury 2000;31(7):479–82.
43. Krywko DM, Toy FK, Mahan ME, et al. Pregnancy Trauma. In: StatPearls. StatPearls. 2022. Available at: http://www.ncbi.nlm.nih.gov/books/NBK430926/. Accessed March 21, 2022.
44. Krywko DM, Yarrarapu SNS, Shunkwiler SM. Kleihauer Betke Test. In: StatPearls. StatPearls. 2022. Available at: http://www.ncbi.nlm.nih.gov/books/NBK430876/. Accessed March 21, 2022.
45. Creanga AA, Syverson C, Seed K, et al. Pregnancy-Related Mortality in the United States, 2011–2013. Obstet Gynecol 2017;130(2):366–73.
46. James Johnston Walker. Ectopic Pregnancy. Clin Obstet Gynecol. 50(1):89–99.
47. Kadasne AR, Mirghani HM. The role of ultrasound in life-threatening situations in pregnancy. J Emerg Trauma Shock 2011;4(4):508–10.
48. Shinde GR, Vaswani BP, Patange RP, et al. Diagnostic Performance of Ultrasonography for Detection of Abruption and Its Clinical Correlation and Maternal and Foetal Outcome. J Clin Diagn Res JCDR 2016;10(8):QC04-QC07.
49. Page N, Roloff K, Modi AP, et al. Management of Placental Abruption Following Blunt Abdominal Trauma. Cureus. 12(9):e10337. doi:
50. Devabhaktuni P, Konkathi AK. Placental abruption an obstetric emergency: management and outcomes in 180 cases. Int J Reprod Contracept Obstet Gynecol 2020;9(8):3188–95.
51. Shevell T, Malone FD. Management of obstetric hemorrhage. Semin Perinatol 2003;27(1):86–104.
52. Committee Opinion No 713. Antenatal Corticosteroid Therapy for Fetal Maturation. ACOG. 2017. Available at: https://www.acog.org/en/clinical/clinical-guidance/committee-opinion/articles/2017/08/antenatal-corticosteroid-therapy-for-fetal-maturation. Accessed June 7, 2022.
53. ACOG Practice Bulletin No. 183. Postpartum Hemorrhage. Obstet Gynecol 2017;130(4):e168–86.
54. Shakur H, Roberts I, Fawole B, et al. Effect of early tranexamic acid administration on mortality, hysterectomy, and other morbidities in women with post-partum haemorrhage (WOMAN): an international, randomised, double-blind, placebo-controlled trial. Lancet 2017;389(10084):2105–16.
55. ACOG Practice Bulletin No. 184. Vaginal Birth After Cesarean Delivery. Obstet Gynecol 2017;130(5):e217–33.
56. Figueiró-Filho EA, Gomez JM, Farine D. Risk Factors Associated with Uterine Rupture and Dehiscence: A Cross-Sectional Canadian Study. Rev Bras Ginecol E Obstetrícia RBGO Gynecol Obstet 2021;43(11):820–5.
57. Ngan Kee WD, Khaw KS. Vasopressors in obstetrics: what should we be using? Curr Opin Anaesthesiol 2006;19(3):238–43.
58. Evans L, Rhodes A, Alhazzani W, et al. Surviving Sepsis Campaign: International Guidelines for Management of Sepsis and Septic Shock 2021. Crit Care Med 2021;49(11):e1063.
59. Wang T, Liao L, Tang X, et al. Effects of different vasopressors on the contraction of the superior mesenteric artery and uterine artery in rats during late pregnancy. BMC Anesthesiol 2021;21(1):185.

60. Campbell TA, Sanson TG. Cardiac arrest and pregnancy. J Emerg Trauma Shock 2009;2(1):34–42.

61. Jeejeebhoy FM, Zelop CM, Lipman S, et al. Cardiac Arrest in Pregnancy: A Scientific Statement From the American Heart Association. Circulation 2015;132(18): 1747–73.

62. Krywko DM, Sheraton M, Presley B. Perimortem Cesarean. In: StatPearls. StatPearls. 2022. Available at: http://www.ncbi.nlm.nih.gov/books/NBK459265/. Accessed March 18, 2022.

63. Alexander AM, Sheraton M, Lobrano S. Perimortem Cesarean Delivery. In: StatPearls. StatPearls. 2022. Available at: http://www.ncbi.nlm.nih.gov/books/ NBK534240/. Accessed June 7, 2022.

64. Preeclampsia and Eclampsia. National Institute of Health. Available at: https:// www.nichd.nih.gov/health/topics/preeclampsia. Accessed March 18, 2022.

65. ACOG Practice Bulletin No. 222. Gestational Hypertension and Preeclampsia. Obstet Gynecol 2020;135(6):e237–60.

66. Roeder HJ, Lopez JR, Miller EC. Ischemic stroke and cerebral venous sinus thrombosis in pregnancy. Handb Clin Neurol 2020;172:3–31.

67. Bryndziar T, Sedova P, Kramer NM, et al. Seizures Following Ischemic Stroke: Frequency of Occurrence and Impact on Outcome in a Long-Term Population-Based Study. J Stroke Cerebrovasc Dis Off J Natl Stroke Assoc 2016;25(1):150–6.

68. Magann EF, Cleveland RS, Dockery JR, et al. Acute Tocolysis for Fetal Distress: Terbutaline Versus Magnesium Sulphate. Aust N Z J Obstet Gynaecol 1993;33(4): 362–4.

Ultrasound in Pregnancy

Samantha A. King, MD, Alexis Salerno, MD, AEMUS-FPD*,
Sarah Sommerkamp, MD

KEYWORDS

- Obstetric ultrasound • Transvaginal ultrasound • Ultrasound in pregnancy
- Ectopic pregnancy • Gestational age measurement • Point of care ultrasound
- Emergency medicine

KEY POINTS

- Transabdominal ultrasound should be attempted before transvaginal.
- To diagnose an intrauterine pregnancy a fetal pole or yolk sac should be visualized.
- Patients who have undergone assisted reproduction are at a higher risk for heterotopic pregnancies.
- The adnexa and right upper quadrant should be imaged if there is clinical concern for ectopic pregnancy.
- Do not rely on the beta-human chorionic gonadotropin and the discriminatory zone to rule out ectopic or to decide when to obtain an ultrasound.
- In patients who are in labor, place the ultrasound transducer over the pelvis to evaluate fetal presentation.

INTRODUCTION

Almost 2% of emergency department (ED) patient visits involve diagnoses related to pregnancy and childbirth.[1] Based on the ACEP 2016 emergency ultrasound guidelines, point of care ultrasound (POCUS) including evaluation of pregnancy is considered an integral skill and within the scope of practice of emergency physicians.[2] Multiple studies have supported the ability of emergency physicians to accurately diagnose intrauterine pregnancy and that the incorporation of POCUS reduces the likelihood of patients returning with ruptured ectopic pregnancies.[2,3] One study in 2015 showed up to a 3 hour decrease in the length of stay for patients who received a transvaginal POCUS evaluation.[4] Another study in 2019, showed a significantly decreased length of stay for patients with first trimester pregnancy who received a transabdominal or transvaginal POCUS evaluation as compared to those who received a radiology department evaluation.[3]

The Authors have nothing to disclose.
Department of Emergency Medicine, University of Maryland School of Medicine, 110 South Paca Street 6th Floor Suite 200, Baltimore, MD 21201, USA
* Corresponding author.
E-mail address: alexis.salerno@som.umaryland.edu

This article describes techniques and imaging findings while assuming the reader has mastered basic POCUS skills. Hands-on ultrasound practice is essential to obtaining proficiency with POCUS techniques.

PROCEDURAL APPROACH
General Ultrasound Approach

Ultrasound is generally considered safe in pregnancy, with no reported harms. However, sonographers should always perform ultrasounds following the principle of "as low as resonably achievable" (ALARA) to minimize any potential risk of harm.[5–7]

There are two general approaches for imaging a pregnancy, the transabdominal (TABUS) and the transvaginal (TVUS) approach. TABUS is typically performed with a curvilinear probe and TVUS is performed with an endocavitary probe. Given the invasive nature and potential discomfort of a TVUS, these authors recommend first attempting to obtain images using the TABUS approach before TVUS regardless of gestational age or beta-human chorionic gonadotropin (β-hCG) level. If an adequate diagnosis and visualization of gynecological-related structures is sufficient, TVUS would be unnecessary.

Transabdominal approach

TABUS is typically initiated with a low-frequency (2 to 5 MHz) curvilinear transducer.[5] TABUS is aided by a full bladder which creates a sonographic window allowing improved visualization of deeper structures such as the uterus. The initial approach is to obtain a sagittal image with the indicator pointing toward the patient's head. Using the bladder as the sonographic window, visualize the uterus. This image is referred to as the *long view of the uterus* with the fundus on the left edge of the screen and the cervix on the right edge, proximal to the vaginal stripe (**Fig. 1**A). The midline of the uterus can be identified by finding the endometrial stripe, a hypoechoic stripe surrounded on either side by isoechoic myometrium. Once the uterus has been identified, sweep (tilting the probe in the scanning plane) through the uterus to identify intrauterine findings or structures. While sweeping through the pelvis, be sure to evaluate for any signs of free fluid, such as a collection of fluid in the Pouch of Douglas or outlining bowel, that may indicate a ruptured ectopic in the correct clinical setting.[8] Visualization of the endometrial stripe and potential IUP may be improved by adjusting the depth. Zoom features on the machine may also improve visualization.

Having completed a sagittal interrogation, rotate the transducer 90° counterclockwise with the transducer marker pointing toward the patient's right side for a *transverse view* (**Fig. 1**B). Again, using the bladder as a sonographic window, sweep through the entire uterus from superior fundus through the cervix looking for any features consistent with an IUP.

Once the uterus has been visualized in both planes, angle the transducer right or left towards either adnexa. Identification of the adnexa can be assisted by locating the iliac vessels-pulsating structures lateral and inferior to the adnexae. Sweep through each adnexa in the transverse and sagittal plane to identify signs consistent with potential ectopic pregnancy (see details below).

Patients who are thin or have a limited visualization of a gestational sac with the curvilinear transducer may benefit from an evaluation with a high-frequency (5 to 12 MHz) linear transducer before proceeding to transvaginal evaluation.[9] This evaluation should still be performed using an OB setting. The higher frequency transducer may allow for better resolution and identification of an IUP. As a trade-off for the higher frequency, the ultrasound beam has decreased penetration, limiting the use of the linear transducer in larger patients. Given the lack of footprint of a linear transducer,

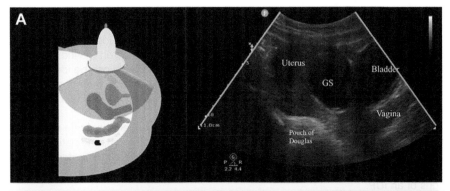

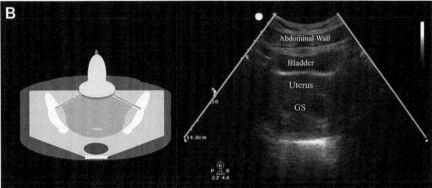

Fig. 1. Transabdominal ultrasound anatomy. This image shows the anatomy for the transabdominal ultrasound technique in the (*A*) sagittal orientation and (*B*) transverse orientation.

these authors still recommend proceeding first with a curvilinear transducer before proceeding to a linear transducer regardless of the patient's body habitus.

If no IUP is visualized or in patients with suspicion for a heterotopic pregnancy, the evaluation should also include imaging of the hepatorenal space to evaluate for free fluid. The sensitivity of this approach can be increased by placing the patient in trendelenburg so that fluid follows gravity and can be visualized in the hepatorenal space. Free fluid in a patient with a pregnancy of unknown location is concerning for a ruptured ectopic pregnancy. Although further imaging may still need to be acquired, identification of findings consistent with a ruptured ectopic may assist in the early mobilization of resources.

Transvaginal Approach
When the initial transabdominal imaging approach does not result in a definitive diagnosis, the patient should undergo transvaginal imaging. Patient positioning is key to the comfort and success of transvaginal imaging. Patients should be placed in the lithotomy position to allow for full range of the transducer throughout imaging. Ideally, patients should empty their bladder before transvaginal imaging to assist in views and comfort.

Before insertion, a small amount of gel followed by sterile cover should be placed on the endocavitary transducer. Additional gel should be used to assist in the insertion of the transducer but is not necessary for visualization due to the mucous membrane environment of the vaginal canal. The endocavitary transducer should be inserted with the transducer marker pointing towards the ceiling to create an image in the *sagittal plane*. Upon insertion, only slight pressure is needed to aid in visualization. In the near field of the ultrasound image, the first visualized structure will be the bladder, if any urine is within it. The uterus should appear just posterior with the fundus on the indicator side traversing the screen to the cervix (**Fig. 2**A). Midline of the uterus can be identified by the hyperechoic endometrial stripe. The operator may need to rock anterior and posterior to center the uterus. Once the midline is located, sweep through the uterus looking for signs of potential IUP or ectopic pregnancy.

After completing a sweep in the sagittal plane, the transducer should be rotated 90 degrees counterclockwise so that the transducer marker is towards the patient's right side creating a *coronal view* (**Fig. 2**B). An additional sweep anterior to posterior should be completed in this plane through the uterus from fundus to cervix, again noting any signs of an IUP.

Once the imaging of the uterus has been completed, the operator should then turn to the adnexa to evaluate for potential signs of ectopic pregnancy. To evaluate the right adnexa, the operator should rock the transducer toward the patient's right by moving the hand holding the transducer towards the patient's left thigh. Once in this plane, the operator should sweep anterior to posterior to interrogate the adnexa, in both the coronal and sagittal plane. The iliac vessels, which should lie posterior and lateral to the ovary, can serve as helpful anatomical landmarks if the operator has difficulty identifying the ovary. Having completed the evaluation of the right adnexa, the endocavitary probe should be directed toward the left adnexa to obtain images in a similar fashion.

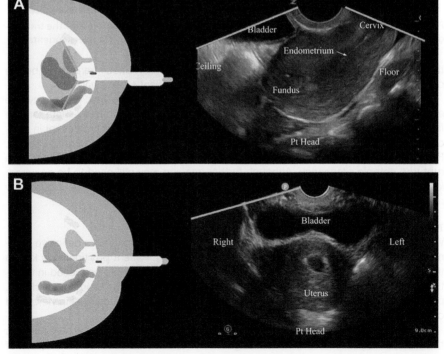

Fig. 2. Transvaginal ultrasound anatomy. This image shows the anatomy for the transvaginal ultrasound technique in the (*A*) sagittal orientation and (*B*) transverse orientation.

DIAGNOSIS OF AN INTRAUTERINE PREGNANCY

The prevailing question for patients presenting to the emergency department and noted to have a positive pregnancy test and pelvic pain or vaginal bleeding is whether the patient has a normally progressing IUP or not. In patients presenting to the emergency department with abdominal pain and/or vaginal bleeding, the identification of an IUP rules out an ectopic pregnancy in patients with low suspicion for a heterotopic pregnancy.[10] The earliest sign, though not yet diagnostic, of intrauterine pregnancy on ultrasound is a gestational sac with the double decidual sac sign.[11] (**Fig. 3**A) This appears a round fluid collection within the uterus with a hyperechoic ring. The gestational sac will typically be observed around 5 weeks gestation. Following the gestational sac, is the identification of a yolk sac, typically visible at 5 to 6 weeks (**Fig. 3**B). Confirmation that the pregnancy is intrauterine occurs only with the identification of a gestational sac and a yolk sac or fetal pole present.[12] The presence of a yolk sac is more specific than a gestational sac alone or a double decidual sac sign. In an ectopic pregnancy, a pseudogestational sac may be present and may be mistaken for a normally developing gestational sac.[13]

In addition to a gestational sac with a yolk sac, this gestational sac must also be surrounded by an endomyometrial mantle of at least 8 mm.[14] Otherwise, consideration for cervical, scar, or interstitial ectopic pregnancy should be considered.

If obtainable, a fetal heart rate (FHR) should be documented. FHR is obtained by identifying a "flickering" in the fetal pole which becomes more apparent as the pregnancy progresses. Place an M-mode cursor through the flickering and obtain an M-mode image. Identify a repeating sinusoidal pattern representing the fetal heartbeat. Using the "calculate FHR" package, the distance between fetal heart beats is measured. Most often, the ultrasound machine will calculate the fetal heart rate using the distance between 2 fetal heart beats. However, the number of fetal heart beats used for calculation can be modified. Embryonic fetal heart rates may vary in the first trimester depending on gestational age.[15] A rate of 110 to 160 bmp is considered normal.[16] (**Fig. 4**). ED providers should not use doppler mode to detect a fetal heartbeat as this increases the power of the ultrasound scan and can therefore increase the potential for biometric effects.

PREGNANCY DATING

Accurate dating in pregnancy is important for patient health outcomes. The most accurate method of dating in pregnancy is an ultrasound performed within the first

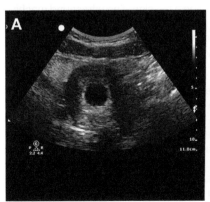
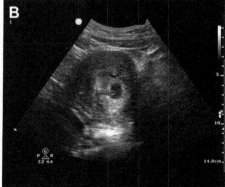

Fig. 3. Normal pregnancy development. (*A*) Double decidual sign. (*B*) Gestational sac with a yolk sac (*arrow*).

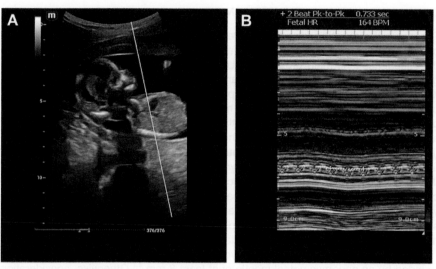

Fig. 4. Fetal heart rate measurement. (*A*) Placement of M-Mode cursor over the fetal heart. (*B*) M-Mode fetal heart tracing with calculation of fetal heart rate.

trimester. The most accurate measurement for dating is a crown-rump-length measurement taken at 8 to 14 weeks of gestational age.[17,18] If a first-trimester ultrasound has been performed, it is recommended that gestational age should not be altered by subsequent second- or third-trimester ultrasounds.[17]

Methods of Dating

Mean sac diameter

The gestational sca is obtained first by locating the pregnancy, then decreasing the depth to maximize the size of the sac on the screen. The operator fans through the ultrasound image to obtain the largest diameter of the gestational sac. If the zoom feature is available, the gestational sac is zoomed in to maximize the accuracy of the measurement. On a frozen image, the height (G1) and the width (G2) is measured to make a "+" sign using the inner wall to inner wall of the gestational sac. Once these calculations are obtained and measurements saved, the transducer is rotated 90 degrees to be orthogonal to the initial view. The image is zoomed and then frozen. In this second image, the length (G3) is measured forming a "−" sign. The ultrasound machine will use these measurements with an appropriate calculation package to give an estimated gestational age. If the ultrasound machine allows, these images can be obtained in "split screen" so that only one image needs to be stored (**Fig. 5**A).

Crown-rump length

For the crown-rump length (CRL) measurement, the pregnancy is located and centered on the ultrasound screen. The size of the pregnancy is maximized on the screen by adjusting the depth of the image. The fetal pole is identified next to the yolk sac within the gestational sac. The operator can then rotate and fan through the image to obtain the maximum length of the fetal pole. Once the maximum length has been found, the image is zoomed in for image optimization. The image is then frozen and the fetal pole is measured from the cephalad to caudal position. The ultrasound calculation package will then calculate an estimated gestational age (**Fig. 5**B). Once a fetal pole is able to flex and extend, this measurement is not as accurate and other measurements should be obtained for estimation of gestational age.[5]

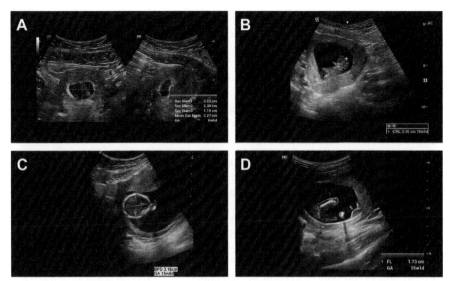

Fig. 5. Gestational age measurements. (*A*) Mean gestational sac diameter, (*B*) crown rump length, (*C*) biparietal diameter, and (*D*) femur length.

Bi-parietal diameter

The Bi-Parietal Diameter (BPD) is measured in the transverse section of the fetal head at the level of the thalami and can be one of the most challenging methods of estimating fetal age. BPD is most commonly used in the late first trimester to about 20 weeks.[5] When measuring the BPD it is important to align the head so that the midline falx and both thalami are visualized. Once positioned correctly, the BPD is measured using the "leading edge to leading edge" technique, or the outer edge of the anterior parietal skull to the inner edge of the posterior parietal skull.[19] The calculation package will then be able to calculate an estimated gestational age (**Fig. 5**C). It may also help to zoom in on the image to obtain a more accurate measurement.

Femur length

Femur length (FL) is more accurate than BPD in late pregnancy and is one of the easiest measurements to obtain.[5] To measure the FL, a still image is obtained with the entire femur in view. The femur length is then measured. This measurement should only include osseous structures in the measurement and exclude any cartilaginous structures. The calculation package will then be able to calculate an estimated gestational age (**Fig. 5**D).

Head circumference

Head circumference (HC) may be the most accurate measurement within the second trimester. The head is aligned so that the midline falx and both thalami are visualized, similar to the BPD measurement.[20] In this plane, the ultrasound software package uses an ellipsoid shape to measure the head circumference.

Abdominal circumference

Abdominal circumference (AC) is obtained by scanning through a fetus in the second or third trimester in the axial plane. The operator identifies the transverse plane in which theportal vein bifurcates. In this plane, the ultrasound software uses an ellipsoid shape to measure the abdominal circumference.

After 14 weeks, it is recommended that the average of BPD, HC, AC, and FL be used for gestational age estimation.[17] In emergency medicine, 2 measurements are traditionally averaged.

DIAGNOSTIC ALGORITHM
Early Pregnancy Algorithm

If a definitive IUP is not identified with point-of-care pelvic ultrasound, further radiologic ultrasound imaging and blood work is recommended to further risk stratify the patient for an ectopic pregnancy (**Fig. 6**).

Limitations of beta-human chorionic gonadotropin levels
One of the blood tests typically obtained in patients with a positive pregnancy test and/or concern for ectopic pregnancy is a quantitative beta-human gonadotropin test (β-hCG). This test can be used in conjunction with an ultrasound or followed serially over time. Discriminatory zones have been cited to guide expected ultrasonography findings of pregnancy. Levels of 1,500 to 2,000 mIU/mL have been cited for detection via transvaginal ultrasound and levels of greater than 5,000 mIU/mL for detection via transabdominal ultrasound.[8]

Regardless of the level of the β-hCG, an ultrasound should be obtained if there is a high clinical concern for ectopic pregnancy.[8,10,21] Ectopic pregnancies have been identified in a wide range of β-hCG levels.[10] Even if the β-hCG level is below the discriminatory zone, an ectopic pregnancy may be present and a level below the threshold should not deter a clinician from obtaining an ultrasound examination.

ULTRASONOGRAPHIC SIGNS OF AN ECTOPIC PREGNANCY

The majority of ectopic pregnancies are located within the fallopian tubes but can alternatively be located in the ovaries, intra-abdominally, cervically, in prior C-section scars, and other locations within the gynecologic tract.[22–24] While an ectopic pregnancy should be suspected in any patient presenting with a positive pregnancy test and no identified IUP on ultrasound, there are key findings that are more suggestive of an ectopic pregnancy. The most definitive but least common of these findings is

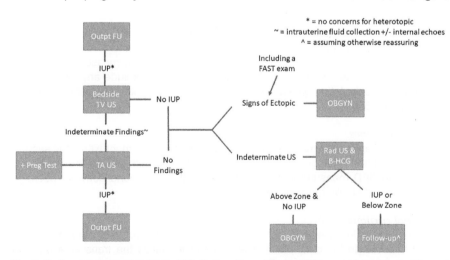

Fig. 6. Early pregnancy algorithm. This figure shows the algorithm used to risk stratify and further work up patients for an ectopic pregnancy.

the presence of an extra-uterine fetal pole, followed by an extrauterine gestational sac with a visualized yolk sac.[8,25] (**Fig. 7**B) More frequently, ectopic pregnancy presents with ultrasound findings of pseudogestational sac, an adnexal mass, ring of fire, or intra-abdominal free fluid.

Pseudogestational Sac

An early gestational sac appears as a fluid collection within the uterus. However, without the presence of a yolk sac, it cannot be definitely diagnosed as an IUP, as it could represent a "pseudogestational sac." An ectopic pregnancy may still develop the fluid collection within the uterus, which can be mistaken to represent an IUP. This fluid collection associated with ectopic pregnancy is called a pseudogestational sac. Pseudogestational sacs will more often have non-rounded shapes and edges. They will also typically lack a double decidual sign (**Fig. 7**A).

As initially noted, although the sac without presence of internal structures is concerning for a pregnancy of unknown location, it may simply represent an early pregnancy.[26,27] Mis-diagnosis of a pseudogestational sac as a normally developing gestational sac in pregnancy is dangerous for potentially missing an ectopic pregnancy but similarly mis-treating a pseudogestational sac as an ectopic pregnancy risks treating a potentially normally developing pregnancy with abortive medication. In clinically stable patients with ultrasound findings of gestational sac versus pseudogestational sac, it is prudent to continue follow-up with serial β-hCG and ultrasounds.[28]

Complex Adnexal Mass

The most common ultrasound finding of an adnexal ectopic pregnancy is an extra-ovarian mass within the adnexa, representing hemorrhage at the site of implantation.[25] There may or may not be surrounding fluid and hypervascularity. The echogenicity and consistency will vary depending on the age of the blood products.[24] (**Fig. 7**C).

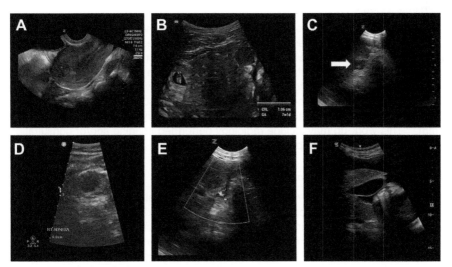

Fig. 7. Signs of ectopic pregnancy. (*A*) Pseudogestational sac. (*B*) Adnexal pregnancy with fetal pole. (*C*) Adnexal Mass (*arrow*). (*D*) Tubal ring. (*E*) Ring of fire. (*F*) Intraperitoneal free fluid in the right upper quadrant.

Tubal Ring/Ring of Fire

The second most common finding of an adnexal ectopic pregnancy is a tubal ring.[24,25] This finding will appear as a "donut" sign within the adnexa (**Fig. 7**D). This ring is the developing gestational sac within the fallopian tube. Given the increased blood flow needed to supply the pregnancy, this area will often be hypervascular, giving a "ring of fire" appearance when color or power doppler is placed over the area.[24] (**Fig. 7**E).

The "ring of fire" can also be found in ovarian cysts and masses, as well as with corpus luteum cysts. Tubal pregnancies will typically be centered within the tissue in comparison to the eccentric corpus luteum cyst.[28] Additionally, tubal rings will appear more echogenic than the surrounding ovarian tissue, while the corpus luteum cyst wall will appear less echogenic. However, it may be difficult to differentiate the two. If there is no confirmed IUP or the patient is at risk for a heterotopic pregnancy, the patient should have further workup for an ectopic pregnancy.

Peritoneal Free Fluid

There may not be definitive findings within the adnexa to diagnose an ectopic pregnancy. Therefore, other signs suggestive of ectopic pregnancy and rupture should be considered. Moderate to large amoubnts of free fluid within the pouch of Douglas is highly suggestive of hemoperitoneum from a ruptured ectopic pregnancy.[25] Physiologic free fluid in the Pouch of Douglas may be present during pregnancy.[24] However, more than a small amount of expected fluid or fluid with debris suggestive of hemorrhage, should raise concern for an ectopic pregnancy.[24] In addition to free fluid within the pelvis, blood from a ruptured ectopic may also collect within the paracolic gutters. Scanning the right upper quadrant may help to more quickly identify a ruptured ectopic and a positive right upper quadrant scan may predict the need for operative intervention.[29] In patients with no findings of IUP on ultrasound and concern for potential ectopic, a right upper quadrant ultrasound should be performed for the evaluation of free fluid (**Fig. 7**F).

Interstitial Ectopic

Interstitial ectopic pregnancies are more rare and occur when there is the implantation of the pregnancy in the interstitium of the fallopian tube.[24] These pregnancies are particularly dangerous with a higher risk of rupture and hemorrhage due to their highly vascular nature, ability to distend, and delayed recognition at later gestational ages.[30] Further diagnostic workup for an interstitial ectopic is warranted with finding of a gestational sac with an endomyometrial mantle measurement less than 8 mm (**Fig. 8**A), though this distance has been cited as varying between 5 mm and 8 mm.[23] This work-up may include radiology performed imaging and/or consultation with obstetrics depending upon institutional practice.

Other Types of Ectopic Pregnancies

It is possible for a pregnancy to implant within the cervical tissue or along a prior cesarean section (C-section) scar.[24,31] Cervical ectopics are diagnosed by the identification of a pregnancy within the cervical tissue, typically lacking the required endomyometrial mantle and lying low within the relative endometrial cavity.[31] C-section ectopic pregnancies will be found along the anterior wall at the site of prior c-section with a decreased endomyometrial mantle measurement.[24] The ED management of these types of ectopic pregnancies are similar and obstetrics consultation should be obtained.

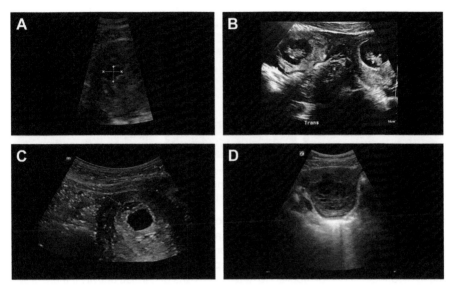

Fig. 8. Abnormal pregnancy findings. (*A*) Cervical ectopic pregnancy. (*B*) Heterotopic pregnancy. (*C*) Arrow: Subchorionic hemorrhage. (*D*) Molar pregnancy.

Heterotopic Pregnancy

A heterotopic pregnancy occurs when there are simultaneous intrauterine and ectopic pregnancies (**Fig. 8**B). The rate of heterotopic pregnancy in the general population is thankfully quite low, estimated to be between 1:4,000 to 1:30,000 for naturally occurring pregnancies.[32] The rate of heterotopic pregnancy increases substantially in individuals who are undergoing reproductive assistance. For these individuals, the rate increases to as high as 1:100.[32] Therefore, it is always important for physicians to ask about reproductive assistance while obtaining patient history. In these situations, the physician should not be complacent after finding an IUP. The adnexa and right upper quadrant should be imaged as well to evaluate for signs of a heterotopic pregnancy.

Intra-abdominal and Ovarian Ectopic Pregnancy

Intra-abdominal ectopic pregnancies and ovarian ectopic pregnancies are unlikely to be diagnosed on ultrasound imaging.[11] Rather, these types of ectopic pregnancies may show signs of hemoperitoneum with rupture, be diagnosed surgically, or through cross-sectional imaging such as MRI.[11]

MISCARRIAGE

It is estimated that about 10% of all clinically recognized pregnancies end in a miscarriage.[33] Patients may present to the ED at different stages of pregnancy loss from missed abortion to complete abortion.

A patient who presents to the ED with vaginal bleeding but no passage of products of conception may have a threatened abortion or a missed abortion.[33] In early pregnancy, if the presence of an ectopic pregnancy has been excluded by imaging, the absence of an embryo in a gestational sac >25 mm, or a blighted ovum, suggests a nonviable pregnancy.[34] (**Fig. 9**A) In a patient where an IUP is identified, there are various nonspecific findings for an abnormal pregnancy that may be revealed on ultrasound imaging. These include fetal bradycardia, low lying gestational sac, abnormal

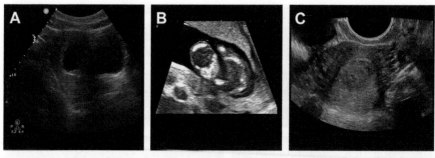

Fig. 9. Signs of miscarriage. (*A*) Large empty gestational sac suggestive of a blighted ovum in a patient with a prior IUP. (*B*) Color Doppler showing no fetal heartbeat. (*C*) Large amount of clot/tissue in endometrium suggestive of an inevitable miscarriage.

size or shape of the gestational sac, and abnormal size or shape of the yolk sac.[34] Embryonic demise is defined as lack of cardiac activity in a fetal pole with CRL > 7 mm.[34] If no heart rate is identified by visualization or M-Mode Doppler, color pulsed Doppler may be used (**Fig. 9**B). Although pulsed Doppler should be avoided during pregnancy due to bioeffects, it can be applied to determine signs of cardiac activity if there is significant concern for fetal demise.[34]

A patient who presents to the ED with vaginal bleeding and passage of products of conception may have a complete miscarriage. On ultrasound, a complete miscarriage is defined as an endometrial thickness <15 mm with no evidence of retained products of conception in a patient who previously was found to have an IUP.[35] Inevitable miscarriages will often have signs of blood clot within the endometrium (**Fig. 9**C).

OTHER EARLY PREGNANCY PATHOLOGY
Subchorionic Hematoma

A subchorionic hematoma is a common finding on routine obstetrical ultrasounds.[36] The hematoma presents as a hypoechoic or anechoic crescent-shaped area behind the gestational sac or fetal membranes(**Fig. 8**C). It may initially appear anechoic, but will have increased echogenicity over time as the blood clots. Though the exact etiology is uncertain, subchorionic hematomas are thought to stem from the detachment of the chorionic membranes from the uterine wall.

The incidence of subchorionic hematomas range from 0.5% to 22%. There are a range of implications from subchorionic hemorrhages. Some studies have shown no effect on pregnancy outcomes, whereas others have shown an increased risk of complications. One meta-analysis showed that subchorionic hematomas statistically increased the rate of spontaneous abortion, abruption, pre-term premature rupture of membranes, and pre-term delivery.[36] There appears to be a relationship between the size and location of the hematoma and rate of complication. Larger hematomas and those located retroplacental portend worse outcomes.[37] It is recommended that women with a subchorionic hematoma visualized in early pregnancy have a repeat ultrasound in 7-10 days.[38]

Molar Pregnancy

Molar pregnancies are grouped under gestational trophoblastic diseases and occur due to abnormal fertilization events.[39] Patients may present to the ED with pelvic pain, vaginal bleeding or hyperemesis and may be found to have an abnormally high β-hCG level.

In a complete molar pregnancy, the classic ultrasound image appears as a cluster of grapes or a snowstorm appearance. The uterus is enlarged with a heterogeneous echogenic mass and several hypoechoic foci creating multiple cystic spaces.[40] (**Fig. 8**D) In a partial molar pregnancy, the ultrasound image will show absent fetal parts and a cystic appearance of the placenta.[40]

SECOND- AND THIRD-TRIMESTER EVALUATION
General Overview

In later term pregnancy, it is important to look for signs of fetal well-being and to evaluate for pathologies that could impact a normal labor process.

Amniotic Fluid Evaluation

Amniotic fluid volume is used to assess for signs of oligohydramnios or polyhydramnios which can relate to a range of pathologies. Two methods for evaluating amniotic fluid volume are the single deepest vertical pocket (SDP) and the amniotic fluid index (AFI).[41,42] The SDP measures the largest vertical diameter of fluid found in the uterine cavity.[41] (**Fig. 10**A) The normal value is 2 cm to 8 cm.[43] The AFI is measured by dividing the uterine cavity into four quadrants. The largest vertical diameter of fluid is measured in each quadrant and added together to obtain the AFI.[41] The normal AFI is 5 cm to 24 cm.[43] (**Fig. 10**B) Studies have shown that AFI may overestimate oligohydramnios and SDP may underestimate.[41] SDP may also overestimate polyhydramnios.[42]

Placenta Previa

Placenta previa occurs when the placenta completely or partially covers the internal cervical os. Placenta previa should be considered in the differential for painless vaginal bleeding in the 3rd trimester. It is important to identify placenta previa, as vaginal examination and progression of labor can increase bleeding or cause hemorrhage.[44]

To evaluate for signs of placenta previa, a transabdominal approach is used to obtain a longitudinal view. If the placenta is visualized at the fundus, there is a low

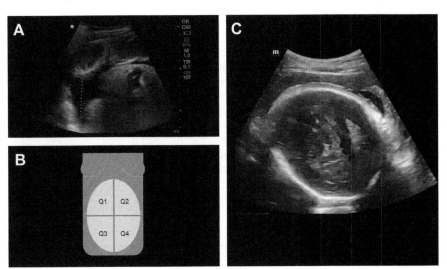

Fig. 10. Late Term Pregnancy Evaluation. (*A*) Measurement of deepest vertical pocket. (*B*) Illustration of four quadrants for obtaining an AFI. (*C*) Fetal head in pelvis.

likelihood of placenta previa. If the placenta is seen near or covering the internal cervical os, placenta previa is of concern and the patient should have further obstetrical imaging.[44] Of note, some cases of placenta previa noted at mid-pregnancy may resolve by the time of delivery.[44]

PLACENTAL ABRUPTION

Placental abruption is a clinical diagnosis with a typical patient presentation of painful vaginal bleeding. Ultrasound has a poor sensitivity for placental abruption and should not be used to exclude the diagnosis. However, there are signs on ultrasound that may suggest placental abruption including pre-placental hematoma collection, increased placental thickness and intra-amniotic hematoma.[45] Patients who have signs of placental abruption on ultrasound have been found to have high maternal morbidity and perinatal mortality.[45]

Fetal Presentation

In a patient who is presenting with signs of labor, it is important to identify the fetal presentation. To evaluate for fetal presentation, the curvilinear transducer is placed transversely over the suprapubic region with the marker towards the patient's right.[46] In a cephalic presentation, the fetal skull will be visualized in the pelvis (**Fig. 10C**). In the term, laboring patient, any fetal part other than the head within the maternal pelvis indicates a breech presentation.

OTHER PATHOLOGY IN THE PREGNANT PATIENT

Ultrasound is critical to the diagnostic work-up of patients presenting to the emergency department with pregnancy-related complaints. Ultrasound may also be the preferred imaging modality for a range of other diagnostic complaints which occur during pregnancy including cardiac disease, cholecystitis, appendicitis and deep vein thrombosis.[5] This is due to the low radiation risk associated with ultrasound, both for the mother and fetus; however, care should be taken to appreciate the anatomical differences that occur throughout the course of a pregnancy when performing ultrasound imaging studies.

SUMMARY

Point of care obstetric ultrasound is an integral tool for the astute emergency physician to improve patient care and departmental flow. Knowledge of the techniques for both transabdominal and transvaginal ultrasounds is essential to appropriately diagnose normal and abnormal pregnancies. Noting the importance of clinical judgment, a working knowledge of the early pregnancy algorithm will assist the clinician with the diagnosis of ectopic pregnancies. Ultrasound can be used to assist in dating, identification of presenting parts, and placental abnormalities. Ultrasound is extremely useful in the point-of-care setting and is a key skill in the provision of high-quality care for pregnant women.

CLINICS CARE POINTS

- Many patients present to the emergency department for complaints related to pregnancy.
- Ergency physcians should look for signs of an ectopic pregnancy in a patient with a positive pregnancy test but an empty uterus.

- When performing a POCUS OB study, it is important to document an estimated gestational age and, if able, a fetal heart rate.
- In late second trimester and third trimester pregnancy evaluate for fetal position and amniontic fluid volume.

REFERENCES

1. Cairns C, Kang K. National hospital ambulatory medical care survey: 2019 emergency department summary tables. National Center for Health Statistics (U.S.); 2022. https://doi.org/10.15620/cdc:115748.
2. Ultrasound Guidelines: Emergency, Point-of-Care and Clinical Ultrasound Guidelines in Medicine. Ann Emerg Med 2017;69(5):e27–54.
3. Beals T, Naraghi L, Grossestreuer A, et al. Point of care ultrasound is associated with decreased ED length of stay for symptomatic early pregnancy. Am J Emerg Med 2019;37(6):1165–8.
4. Panebianco NL, Shofer F, Fields JM, et al. The utility of transvaginal ultrasound in the ED evaluation of complications of first trimester pregnancy. Am J Emerg Med 2015;33(6):743–8.
5. Ma OJ, Mateer JR, Reardon RF, et al. Emergency ultrasound, Fourth Edition, McGraw Hill; New York.
6. Reddy UM, Abuhamad AZ, Levine D, et al. Fetal imaging: Executive Summary of a Joint Eunice Kennedy Shriver National Institute of Child Health and Human Development, Society for Maternal-Fetal Medicine, American Institute of Ultrasound in Medicine, American College of Obstetricians and Gynecologists, American College of Radiology, Society for Pediatric Radiology, and Society of Radiologists in Ultrasound Fetal Imaging Workshop. Am J Obstet Gynecol 2014;210(5):387–97.
7. Bagley J, Thomas K, DiGiacinto D. Safety Practices of Sonographers and Their Knowledge of the Biologic Effects of Sonography. J Diagn Med Sonogr 2011; 27(6):252–61.
8. Baker M, dela Cruz J. Ectopic Pregnancy, Ultrasound. In: StatPearls [Internet]. Treasure Island FL: StatPearls Publishing; 2022.
9. Tabbut M, Harper D, Gramer D, et al. High-frequency linear transducer improves detection of an intrauterine pregnancy in first-trimester ultrasonography. Am J Emerg Med 2016;34(2):288–91.
10. Hahn SA, Promes SB, Brown MD, et al. Clinical Policy: Critical Issues in the Initial Evaluation and Management of Patients Presenting to the Emergency Department in Early Pregnancy. Ann Emerg Med 2017;69(2):241–50.e20.
11. Scibetta EW, Han CS. Ultrasound in Early Pregnancy. Obstet Gynecol Clin North Am 2019;46(4):783–95.
12. Herbst MK, Tafti D, Shanahan MM. Obstetric Ultrasound. In: StatPearls [Internet]. StatPearls Publishing. Treasure Island (FL) 2022.
13. Nyberg DA, Mack LA, Harvey D, et al. Value of the yolk sac in evaluating early pregnancies. J Ultrasound Med 1988;7(3):129–35.
14. Lewiss RE, Shaukat NM, Saul T. The endomyometrial thickness measurement for abnormal implantation evaluation by pelvic sonography. J Ultrasound Med Off J Am Inst Ultrasound Med 2014;33(7):1143–6.
15. Doubilet PM, Benson CB. Embryonic heart rate in the early first trimester: what rate is normal? J Ultrasound Med 1995;14(6):431–4.

16. Pildner von Steinburg S, Boulesteix AL, Lederer C, et al. What is the "normal" fetal heart rate? PeerJ 2013;1:e82.

17. Methods for estimating the due date. Committee Opinion No. 700. American College of Obstetricians and Gynecologists. Obstet Gynecol, 129, 2017, e150–e154.

18. O'Gorman N, Salomon LJ. Fetal biometry to assess the size and growth of the fetus. Best Pract Res Clin Obstet Gynaecol 2018;49:3–15.

19. Salerno A, Flanagan K, Ghaffarian K, et al. of Emergency Physician Performed Biparietal Diameter Estimate for Gestational Age. J Emerg Med 2022;62(3): 342–7.

20. Skinner C, Mount CA. Sonography assessment of gestational age. In: StatPearls [Internet]. StatPearls Publishing. Treasure Island (FL) 2022.

21. Kadar N, Bohrer M, Kemmann E, et al. The discriminatory human chorionic gonadotropin zone for endovaginal sonography: a prospective, randomized study. Gynecol Endocrinol 1994;61(6):1016–20.

22. Bouyer J. Sites of ectopic pregnancy: a 10 year population-based study of 1800 cases. Hum Reprod 2002;17(12):3224–30.

23. Doane B, Perera P. Emergency Ultrasound Identification of a Cornual Ectopic Pregnancy. West J Emerg Med 2012;13(4):315.

24. Lee R, Dupuis C, Chen B, et al. Diagnosing ectopic pregnancy in the emergency setting. Ultrasonography 2018;37(1):78–87.

25. Dialani V, Levine D. Ectopic Pregnancy: A Review. Ultrasound Q 2004;20(3):13.

26. Lee IT, Rubin ES, Wu J, et al. The incidence and importance of the pseudogestational sac revisited. Am J Obstet Gynecol 2022;226(4):537.e1–7.

27. Phillips CH, Benson CB, Durfee SM, et al. "Pseudogestational Sac" and Other 1980s-Era Concepts in Early First-Trimester Ultrasound: Are They Still Relevant Today? J Ultrasound Med 2020;39(8):1547–51.

28. Bolaji I, Singh M, Goddard R. Sonographic Signs in Ectopic Pregnancy: Update. Ultrasound 2012;20(4):192–210.

29. Rodgerson JD, Heegaard WG, Plummer D, et al. Emergency department right upper quadrant ultrasound is associated with a reduced time to diagnosis and treatment of ruptured ectopic pregnancies. Acad Emerg Med 2001;8(4):331–6.

30. Lin EP. Diagnostic clues to ectopic pregnancy. Radiographics 2008;28(6): 1661–71.

31. Modayil V, Ash A, Raio C. Cervical ectopic pregnancy diagnosed by point-of-care emergency department ultrasound. J Emerg Med 2011;41(6):655–7.

32. Committee on Practice Bulletins—Gynecology. ACOG Practice Bulletin No. 191: Tubal Ectopic Pregnancy. Obstet Gynecol 2018;131(2):e65–77.

33. Dugas C, Slane VH. Miscarriage. StatPearls Publishing. 2022. Available at: https://www.ncbi.nlm.nih.gov/books/NBK532992/. Accessed June 6, 2022.

34. Brown DL, Packard A, Maturen KE, et al. ACR Appropriateness Criteria ® First Trimester Vaginal Bleeding. J Am Coll Radiol 2018;15(5):S69–77.

35. Jauniaux E, Johns J, Burton GJ. The role of ultrasound imaging in diagnosing and investigating early pregnancy failure. Ultrasound Obstet Gynecol 2005;25(6): 613–24.

36. Tuuli MG, Norman SM, Odibo AO, et al. Perinatal outcomes in women with subchorionic hematoma: a systematic review and meta-analysis. Obstet Gynecol 2011;117(5):1205–12.

37. Hashem A, Sarsam SD. The Impact of Incidental Ultrasound Finding of Subchorionic and Retroplacental Hematoma in Early Pregnancy. J Obstet Gynecol India 2019;69(1):43–9.

38. American College of Obstetricians and Gynecologists' Committee on Practice Bulletins—Gynecology. ACOG Practice Bulletin No. 200: Early Pregnancy Loss. Obstet Gynecol. 132(5), 2018, e197-e207.

39. Horowitz NS, Eskander RN, Adelman MR, et al. Epidemiology, diagnosis, and treatment of gestational trophoblastic disease: A Society of Gynecologic Oncology evidenced-based review and recommendation. Gynecol Oncol 2021; 163(3):605–13.

40. Lok C, Frijstein M, van Trommel N. Clinical presentation and diagnosis of Gestational Trophoblastic Disease. Best Pract Res Clin Obstet Gynaecol 2021;74: 42–52.

41. Kehl S, Schelkle A, Thomas A, et al. Single deepest vertical pocket or amniotic fluid index as evaluation test for predicting adverse pregnancy outcome (SAFE trial): a multicenter, open-label, randomized controlled trial. Ultrasound Obstet Gynecol 2016;47(6):674–9.

42. Hughes DS, Magann EF, Whittington JR, et al. Accuracy of the Ultrasound Estimate of the Amniotic Fluid Volume (Amniotic Fluid Index and Single Deepest Pocket) to Identify Actual Low, Normal, and High Amniotic Fluid Volumes as Determined by Quantile Regression. J Ultrasound Med 2020;39(2):373–8.

43. Indications for outpatient antenatal fetal surveillance. ACOG Committee Opinion No. 828. American College of Obstetricians and Gynecologists. Obstet Gynecol. 137, 2021, e177–e197.

44. Silver RM. Abnormal Placentation: Placenta Previa, Vasa Previa, and Placenta Accreta. Obstet Gynecol 2015;126(3):654–68.

45. Shinde GR, Vaswani BP, Patange RP, et al. Diagnostic Performance of Ultrasonography for Detection of Abruption and Its Clinical Correlation and Maternal and Foetal Outcome. J Clin Diagn Res JCDR 2016;10(8):QC04-07.

46. Youssef A, Ghi T, Pilu G. How to perform ultrasound in labor: assessment of fetal occiput position. Ultrasound Obstet Gynecol 2013;41(4):476–8.

Pediatric and Adolescent Gynecologic Emergencies

Marissa Wolfe, MD[a], Emily Rose, MD[b],*

KEYWORDS

- Vulvovaginitis • Pelvic inflammatory disease • Ovarian torsion • Straddle injuries
- Sexually transmitted infections • Inguinal hernia

KEY POINTS

- Prepubescent children have unique pathophysiology secondary to a lack of estrogen including noncandidal vulvovaginitis, labial adhesions, and urethral prolapse.
- Ovarian torsion most frequently occurs with an ovarian mass but may occur in prepubescent girls with normal ovaries secondary to a hypermobile adnexa.
- Sexually transmitted infections are common in adolescence and warrant screening and treatment to minimize long-term complications including infertility and chronic pain.

INTRODUCTION

Pediatric gynecology encompasses a range of topics and unique issues to childhood. These conditions present at various developmental and hormonal stages in young childhood and adolescence. There are also specific challenges in caring for an adolescent who is developing independence and making choices independent of parental oversight. This article reviews normal physiology in children, common pathophysiology unique to children in the prepubertal period, as well as common injuries and infections of the genitourinary system.

EXAMINATION

The gynecologic examination of pediatric patients in the emergency department requires age-appropriate consideration and adjustment depending on the involved circumstances. Care must be taken to avoid a traumatic experience for a child. Communication before and during the examination about each step of the examination

[a] Los Angeles County + University of Southern California Medical Center, 1200 North State Street, Room 1060E, Los Angeles, CA 90033, USA; [b] Pre-Health Undergraduate Studies, Department of Emergency Medicine, Keck School of Medicine of the University of Southern California, Los Angeles County + University of Southern California Medical Center, Old General Hospital, 1200 North State Street, Room 1100, Los Angeles, CA 90033, USA
* Corresponding author.
E-mail address: emilyros@usc.edu

Emerg Med Clin N Am 41 (2023) 355–367
https://doi.org/10.1016/j.emc.2023.01.006
0733-8627/23/© 2023 Elsevier Inc. All rights reserved.

is important. Specific examination techniques for the evaluation of a young child include the frog-leg position (legs flexed and abducted at the hips) or the knee-chest position. In the frog-leg position, the child may either lay on the gurney or sit in a caregiver's lap. The knee-chest position may also be used. In this position, the child lays pronated with her weight on her knees, and her buttock elevated.

In most cases of prepubertal girls, only external evaluation should be performed in the emergency department. If an internal examination is warranted, the examination should be performed under sedation.

Adolescents have legal protection to their privacy regarding sexual and reproductive health care. They are more likely to share specific details if confidentiality is ensured.

NORMAL ANATOMY
Neonate

Neonatal anatomy differs from older children. In utero estrogen exposure causes many gynecologic differences between neonates and older infants. Estrogen levels typically influence anatomy for the first 6 months of life, and levels steadily fall until around 2 years of age. Estrogen may cause the labia majora, labia minora, and clitoris to appear full or enlarged. The normal clitoral width is 2 to 6 mm, length varies but is typically less than 9 mm.[1] The clitoris is fully developed by 27 weeks so it may seem relatively large in preterm infants with less labial fat. An abnormally large clitoris may be caused by congenital adrenal hyperplasia, androgen-secreting tumors, or androgen insensitivity in a genetic male. The labia majora is also not distinct from the labia minora in neonates. The labia majora may seem hyperpigmented, and a thick, redundant hymen may also be noted. Breast buds may also be present in young infants.

Additionally, physiologic discharge and bleeding may be present from in utero estrogen exposure within the first 2 to 3 weeks of life. Vaginal discharge may be white, yellow, and/or mucoid. Bleeding may also occur.[2]

Vaginal skin tags and hymenal skin tags may also be present on examination. These are considered normal variants and will spontaneously regress without intervention.

Infancy to Adolescence

Prepubertal vaginal mucosa is thin and redder than in adolescence. With puberty, estrogen stimulation thickens the vaginal mucosa to a dull-pink mucoid surface. During puberty, a thin discharge may be present. This is normal as long as it is not purulent or foul smelling. Foul smelling discharge or bleeding before the onset of puberty should trigger concern for retained foreign body or sexual abuse.

There are disease processes that may present with precocious or delayed puberty. Precocious puberty is defined as breast development before the age of 8 years, and late puberty is defined as breast development after the age of 12 to 13. The causes of abnormal pubertal development in a child include idiopathic conditions, nutritional deficiencies, hypothalamic-pituitary-gonadal axis variations, or neoplastic and genetic disorders. Ambiguous genitalia should be referred for further genetic testing. A review of the Tanner stages can be seen in **Fig. 1**.

The evaluation of the hymen is an important aspect of evaluation for potential sexual abuse. It is important to note that the vast majority of girls who have been sexually assaulted have a normal genital examination. Accidental injury typically spares the hymen. Any hymenal injury particularly in the posterior portion (4–8 o'clock) is highly concerning for penetrating trauma. Additionally, anatomic variants are common,

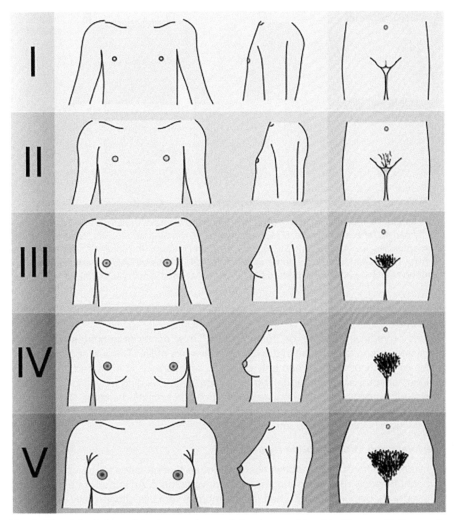

Fig. 1. Visual depiction of the tanner stages of development in girls. (*Source*: M. Komornic-zak, https://commons.wikimedia.org/w/index.php?curid=7121327.)

which may be mistaken for abuse. The appearance of the hymen changes with age. Newborns have a thick hymen with a prominent ridge at the 6 o'clock position. Mucus or bleeding may be present stimulated by maternal estrogen. In older prepubertal girls, the lack of estrogen makes the hymen thin with many different variants including annular, posterior rim, redundant, cribriform, imperforate, and microperforate (**Fig. 2**).[3] During puberty, the hymen thickens with estrogen stimulation.

PATHOLOGIC CONDITIONS
Neonatal Vaginal Bleeding

Blood noted inside of a diaper is a commonly encountered presenting concern. Red color in the diaper may be from the urine, vagina, or stool. Urate crystals can mimic the appearance of blood. Urate crystals are orange-red in color and are present in

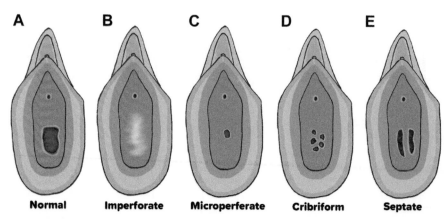

Fig. 2. Variations in hymen anatomy. (*A*) Normal hymen, (*B*) Imperforate hymen, (*C*) Microperforate hymen, (*D*) cribiform hymen, (*E*) Septate hymen. (*From* Guyther Jennifer. Pediatric Female GU Emergencies. In: Mattu A and Swadron S, ed. CorePendium. Burbank, CA: CorePendium, LLC. https://www.emrap.org/corependium/chapter/rec4a1zbbVdbuTy4R/Pediatric-Female-GU-Emergencies#h.3wyg2ojktdyl. Updated May 7, 2021. Accessed January 6, 2023.)

highly concentrated urine, especially in the first few days of life when breast milk volume is low.

Cases of vaginal bleeding, or "mini-menses," may occur as neonates have withdrawal from prenatal estrogen in the first 2 to 3 weeks of life. This will spontaneously resolve without intervention, and only caregiver reassurance is indicated. If bleeding continues beyond 3 weeks, further workup is required. Bleeding may also be present in the stool secondary to maternal cracked nipples in breastfed infants. Due to rapid gut transit time, this may seem bright red in the stool. An examination of the mother typically reveals this as the source of bleeding.[4]

Imperforate and Microperforate Hymens

The hymen is a fibrous, connective tissue structure that attaches to the vaginal walls and spontaneously ruptures during neonatal development. An imperforate hymen, or microperforate hymen, occurs when this membrane remains either totally or partially intact and may cause obstructive symptoms within the vaginal canal as mucus or blood accumulates proximally.[3] An imperforate hymen may present during the neonatal period with a bulging membrane secondary to mucus production stimulated by maternal estrogen. If unrecognized in the neonatal period, it presents during menarche when blood accumulates in the vaginal canal. Hematocolpos (accumulation of blood proximal to the hymen) may present as a blueish discoloration behind the vaginal membrane. This obstruction may lead to cyclical abdominal pain and may have associated lower abdominal mass, urinary retention, or constipation.

The diagnosis of imperforate hymen is confirmed by visual external examination. Treatment is a definitive hymenectomy performed under anesthesia by a pediatric gynecologist or general surgeon. Urgent intervention may be required with more severe symptoms such as associated acute urinary retention.

Urethral Prolapse

Urethral prolapse is a rare condition, which occurs in prepubertal girls aged 2 to 10 years. It is typically asymptomatic, and occurs when the distal portion of the urethra protrudes through the external urethral meatus, resulting in a circumferential, "doughnut-shaped," mass at the urethral opening. Partial prolapse can also occur either anteriorly or posteriorly. Urethral prolapse is typically painless, although less commonly can be associated with scant bleeding, dysuria, or urinary retention. The prolapsed urethral tissue is friable and may rarely become infected or even necrose. The most common presentation is when parents note blood/spotting in a young girl's underwear. It is more common in girls of African-American descent and occurs secondary to low estrogen production. It can also be associated with increased intra-abdominal pressure, such as in cases of constipation or secondary to other preceding events, such as local trauma.[5]

Although a benign finding that is typically incidentally found, it is important to consider a broad differential to rule out other causes including a sarcoma botryoides, prolapsed ureterocele, periurethral abscess, vaginal or cervical prolapse, and rhabdomyosarcoma. Once the diagnosis is confirmed, treatment includes topical estrogen therapy applied to the prolapsed tissue twice a day. Evaluation for resolution should occur after 2 weeks of treatment. Most prolapses respond after 2 weeks of treatment but sometimes longer courses of therapy are indicated. Sitz baths twice daily may also facilitate resolution. Additionally, straining should be avoided by providing an appropriate bowel regimen in cases of constipation. Manual reduction of the prolapse is not required and should not be attempted. Urologist should be consulted if there is any evidence of significant bleeding, necrosis, or thrombosis. Follow-up with the patient's primary pediatrician should be obtained in 1 to 2 weeks, with consideration for a urology referral outpatient in refractory cases.

Labial Adhesion

Labial adhesions are typically incidentally found by caretakers in infants aged between 3 months and 3 years. They occur when the labia minora fuse in the presence of inflammation and a low-estrogen environment. A grayish fibrotic membrane joins the labia and is referred to as "raphe" at the point of fusion. Adhesions may be partial, involving either the upper or lower labia, or complete with only a small orifice allowing urine to be expelled. Common causes include local trauma, poor perineal hygiene, infection, or other inflammatory processes such as Steven Johnson syndrome, lichen sclerosis, graft versus host disease, or Behcet disease. Because local trauma may be a preceding event, sexual abuse should also be considered.

Although most labial adhesions are asymptomatic, patients may present with abnormal voiding, urinary frequency, postvoid dribbling, abnormal discharge, or dysuria. For asymptomatic patients, proper hygiene should be emphasized and no further treatment is indicated, and adhesions typically resolve during puberty. If patients are symptomatic, topical medications may be used. The risks versus benefits of medications should be discussed with parents before initiating treatment. The most common topical medication used is estrogen, which may be applied to the affected area (the point of midline fusion where there is a thin, white line) twice daily for 2 to 6 weeks. Parents should be warned that this treatment may cause local irritation, vulvar hyperpigmentation, breast bud formation, and mild vaginal bleeding. These symptoms resolve after cessation of the topical estrogen cream.[5] If estrogen treatment fails, topical betamethasone can be offered twice daily for 4 to 6 weeks as a second-line therapy. Prolonged topical steroid use (>3 months) may result in skin atrophy and systemic corticosteroid absorption. Manual or surgical separation of the labia is rarely indicated and typically only performed in those with severe urinary obstruction. Larger, thicker adhesions are more likely to be resistant to topical therapy and require separation by a specialist. Topical estrogen cream is recommended after separation to prevent recurrence.

Vulvovaginitis

Vulvovaginitis is a common gynecologic complaint in children. Prepubescent girls are particularly at risk due to a low-estrogen environment leading to sensitive and thin epithelium, poor hygiene, and susceptible anatomy. Girls have a close physical distance between the anus and the vulva, a neutral vaginal pH, and lack labial fat pads and hair, which puts them at higher risk for vulvovaginitis. This combination of factors, as well as exacerbation by chemical irritants found in soaps or lotions or tight, nonbreathable clothing, can cause worsening local irritation.

Patients typically present with irritation, discomfort, mucoid discharge, itching, erythema, rash, and dysuria. The examination will be notable for erythema and scant discharge or bleeding may be present. Associated bacterial infection, retained vaginal foreign body, or sexual abuse should be considered. Bacterial infections or foreign bodies typically have more copious, foul-smelling discharge. Evidence of trauma and abnormalities of the hymen such as tears or posterior notching should be noted, especially in potential cases of sexual abuse.

Although most cases are nonspecific and secondary to local irritation, there are many possible infectious pathogens that may contribute to symptoms. Self-inoculation with respiratory pathogens such as *Streptococcus pyogenes* or *Haemophilus influenzae* may occur. *S pyogenes* infections most commonly occur from autoinoculation and appear "beefy red" in the perineal region, or frequently perianal as well. Additionally, many enteric pathogens may grow on vaginal culture. Sexually transmitted infections (STIs) such as *Neisseria gonorrhoeae* or *Chlamydia trachomatis* often have associated yellow or green discharge but may rarely be asymptomatic. Identification of these organisms should trigger investigation for abuse. Candida occurs in only a very small percentage of prepubertal girls. Pinworms should also be considered with perianal and vulvar irritation with severe pruritus.

Treatment is primarily focused on improving hygiene and removing irritants such as bubble baths or tight clothing. Daily bathing with gentle soap only is recommended. After baths, patients should rinse the vagina with water to remove any soap residue. Toilet hygiene is also important. Young girls can sit backward on the toilet with their legs separated to minimize urine reflux into the vagina. Additionally, patients and parents should be counseled on front-to-back wiping to minimize stool contamination of the perineal area. Sitz baths and barrier cream should also be considered to minimize exposure to irritants.

Most vulvovaginitis responds to hygiene treatment alone. In refractory or worsening cases, a 10-day course of amoxicillin or amoxicillin-clavulanate oral therapy, or topical clindamycin or metronidazole can be considered. Infections with *S pyogenes* frequently require antibiotic therapy. Infections with *Yersinia* are also typically resistant to hygiene treatment alone. A repeat examination should be performed if a patient returns to the emergency department to again evaluate for a foreign body in refractory cases.[6]

Vulvovaginitis may be accompanied by dysuria. When it is, a urine dipstick should be performed to evaluate for a urinary tract infection. A clean catch urine specimen is often difficult in this age group and vaginitis can cause small numbers of WBC and RBC in the urine. A urinary culture may help delineate a true urinary tract infection from a contaminated specimen.

Vaginal Foreign Body

A vaginal foreign body may cause acute or chronic recurrent vulvovaginitis. Children present with vaginal discharge, intermittent bleeding, and/or a foul-smelling odor. Toilet paper is the most commonly encountered foreign body but other small objects such as toys, hair ties, and common household items may be found. Button batteries may cause local necrosis and often have associated gray, watery discharge.

The diagnosis of vaginal foreign body is suspected on history and confirmed with visual inspection. The knee to chest position facilitates visualization. Vaginoscopy may be required, which frequently requires sedation.

Removal can be facilitated by gentle irrigation with warm normal saline using a syringe connected to an infant Foley catheter or feeding tube. Topical lidocaine jelly may be used to facilitate the procedure. The catheter should be lubricated and inserted 1 to 2 cm into the vagina with approximately 200 mL of saline injected slowly until objects removed.[6] If unsuccessful or another object is suspected, gynecologic examination under anesthesia with a pediatric gynecologist is indicated.

Button batteries may cause deep vaginal burns or perforation, so removal under sedation is indicated followed by inspection for associated damage with vaginoscopy. Severe burns may involve damage to the bladder or rectal mucosa.

Ovarian Torsion

Ovarian torsion is a surgical emergency that mandates consideration in any female patient with abdominal or pelvic pain. Torsion may occur at any age, including in a fetus in utero but is most common during childbearing years. Torsion occurs when blood flow is obstructed secondary to twisting of an ovary on the ligaments that typically hold it in place. Although many patients have an abnormality of the ovary that leads to twisting, such as a cyst, in infants and prepubescent girls, a physiologically normal ovary may still torse secondary to a hypermobile, long, fallopian tube, mesosalpinx, or mesoovarium.

Risk factors for torsion include prior torsion and an ovarian mass. The most common predisposing factor for torsion is an ovarian cyst or benign neoplasm. More than 85% of ovarian torsion is associated with an ovarian mass. Lesions greater than 5 cm are more likely to torse, and there is no established upper limit of size, which makes torsion less likely (lesions >30 cm have been described to cause torsion). Fixed lesions (eg. malignant) are less likely to torse. The right ovary tends to torse more commonly than the left. This is likely secondary to a longer utero-ovarian ligament on the right and the stabilizing presence of the sigmoid colon on the left.

Signs and symptoms of torsion are often nonspecific but most commonly include unilateral pain and vomiting. More than 90% of patients have moderate-to-severe pelvic pain that may be described as sharp, stabbing, dull, cramping, or colicky. Radiation of pain to the flank, back, or groin may be present. Frequently, there is a history of recent vigorous activity. Laboratory testing is additionally nonspecific, although pregnancy testing should be obtained. Diagnosis can be supported using ultrasound with Doppler, although ultrasound is not entirely sensitive (43%–75%).[7,8] Doppler flow may be normal, decreased, or absent in a torsed ovary due to intermittent or incomplete torsion or due to collateral blood supply. Findings may include an enlarged, edematous ovary on ultrasound, the presence of an adnexal mass, diminished flow on color Doppler, displacement of the ovary and uterus, or free fluid in the pelvis. The presence of a whirlpool sign indicates the twisting of vessels secondary to twisting of the ovarian pedicle. Venous compression may also be seen. Absence of arterial flow occurs only in 40% to 73%. A high index of suspicion is necessary because all diagnostics may be normal, and torsion carries a risk of ovarian necrosis and subsequent infertility. Torsion should be suspected in recurrent and paroxysm of pain even if the ultrasound is unremarkable. Definitive diagnosis of torsion is made by visual inspection during surgical exploration.

All patients with suspected torsion require emergent evaluation by a pediatric surgeon or a gynecologist for possible surgical intervention. The surgical intervention of choice, if possible, is detorsion rather than oophorectomy because even necrotic-appearing ovaries may remain viable.[9] The dusky appearance is often secondary to vascular and lymphatic congestion rather than true necrosis because the total arterial occlusion often does not occur. Because of this, prolonged time of symptoms does not preclude ovarian salvage.[10] Ischemic torsion may be more likely with elevated inflammatory markers, such as elevated WBC and elevated C-reactive protein (CRP), and vomiting.[11] Oophoropexy may be performed in recurrent torsion or in patients with one remaining ovary.

If torsion is undiagnosed and untreated, necrosis of the ovarian and adnexal tissue will occur. This tissue may involute or autoamputate and have associated scarring. In addition to the most common and concerning complication of infertility, adhesions may cause chronic pelvic pain. Severe hemorrhage and peritonitis are uncommon during acute torsion but may rarely occur.

Inguinal Hernias

Infants are at risk for inguinal hernias due to a short inguinal canal, which aligns internal and external inguinal rings. Premature infants with increased intra-abdominal pressure from mechanical ventilation are at particular risk. The incidence is 4 times higher in male infants. In female infants, hernias contain the suspensory ligament of the ovary so many hernias also contain the ovary and/or fallopian tube. Ovarian torsion within a hernia is well described.[12] Rarely, hernias may even contain the uterus.

Inguinal hernias typically presents as a nonpainful, reducible mass. When hernias are irreducible, an incarcerated or strangulated hernia should be considered and diagnostic ultrasound performed. Emergency surgical consultation is indicated if there is evidence of incarceration, strangulation, ovarian torsion, or necrosis. Other cases may be referred for surgical correction on an outpatient basis.

Straddle Injuries

Straddle injuries are caused by direct trauma to the groin, genitalia, or perineum. The trauma may be blunt or penetrating. In blunt trauma, injury is sustained by compressive forces against the bony margins of the pelvic outlet. Most straddle injuries are anterior or lateral to the hymen and involve the mons, clitoral hood, and the labia minora. Hematomas and superficial lacerations are more common with blunt injury and less commonly require intervention.

Penetrating injuries occur when a child is impaled by an object and are typically more severe and extensive. These injuries may be associated with peritoneal perforation, urethral disruption, or rectal injury. Examination findings indicating more serious injury include evidence of injury to the hymen or posterior fourchette, perineal lacerations, or blood at the urethral meatus. Deep vaginal and vulvar lacerations that extend into the posterior cul-de-sac may cause severe hemorrhage and hemodynamic instability.

Although most straddle injuries affect superficial tissue only, the involvement of the internal and external pudendal artery can cause more significant bleeding. Large vulvar hematomas may cause urinary obstruction. Additionally, the vulvar tissue is friable and often associated with significant bleeding. A vaginal laceration should be suspected if bleeding occurs from the introitus. Evaluation with sedation is necessary to facilitate examination and repair of the laceration. Sexual abuse should always be considered with this kind of injury, and special attention should be paid to ensure that the mechanism of injury matches the injury pattern. Other findings suspicious of sexual abuse include lacerations of the hymen, posterior fourchette, and lateral vaginal walls. Any hymenal injury in the 3 o'clock to 9 o'clock position is consistent

Table 1
Most common presentations of sexually transmitted infections

Disease	Clinical Presentation and Specific Features
C trachomatis + *N gonorrhoeae* cervicitis and urethritis	Most cases are asymptomatic. Cervicitis: • Mucopurulent discharge • Easily induced endocervical bleeding ○ May present as intermenstrual vaginal bleeding or postcoital bleeding • Edematous cervical ectopy Urethritis: (occurs in approximately 15% of cervicitis) • Dysuria • Urinary frequency
Bacterial vaginosis	Not classified as sexually transmitted infection but sexual activity is a risk factor Vaginosis: • Off-white, thin, homogeneous discharge • "Fishy smell"
Trichomoniasis	Often asymptomatic Vaginitis: • Vulvar and vaginal mucosa erythema Cervicitis: • Green-yellow, frothy discharge • Malodorous • Strawberry cervix"—punctate hemorrhages of vaginal wall and cervix

Syphilis	• Primary: Chancre—painless, single papule
	  ○ Papule ulcerates with a raised, indurated, well-circumscribed margin
	  ○ Mild bilateral lymphadenopathy
	• Secondary:
	  ○ Constitutional symptoms
	  ○ Adenopathy
	  ○ Maculopapular or pustular rash with palm and sole involvement
	  ○ Condylomata lata—large, raised, gray-white lesions
	  ○ Alopecia
	  ○ Gastrointestinal, liver, renal, neurologic, ocular, or musculoskeletal involvement
	• Late
	  ○ Cardiovascular or central nervous system involvement
	  ○ Gummatous lesions

Genital herpes	• Painful, multiple, bilateral lesions • Begin as grouped vesicles on an erythematous base • Open into shallow ulcerations • May have systemic symptoms (fever, myalgias)
Lymphogranuloma venereum (*C trachomatis*)	• Painless, single ulcer or papules • May have systemic symptoms • Delayed lymphadenopathy—matted, painful lymph nodes possible

(continued on next page)

Table 1 (continued)	
Disease	**Clinical Presentation and Specific Features**
	• Anorectal symptoms may concomitantly occur with rectal discharge, pain, bleeding, tenesmus, and constipation
Chancroid (*Haemophilus ducreyi*)	• Painful, multiple lesions • Erythematous papules, pustules that ulcerate • Deep, ragged ulcerations with purulent yellow-gray base and undermined, violaceous border • Lymphadenopathy—matted, painful lymph nodes possible
Granuloma inguinale (*Klebsiella granulomatis*)	• Painless, single or multiple lesions • Nodules that ulcerate with raised, rolling margins • Friable
HIV	• Constitutional symptoms • Adenopathy • Oropharyngeal findings • Generalized, nonspecific rash • Gastrointestinal, respiratory, neurologic symptoms • Opportunistic infections

with a penetration injury. Other findings suggestive of unintentional injury include a single or stellate laceration.

Treatment involved depends on the injury sustained. Hematomas involving the labia, mons, and clitoris can be managed conservatively with cold compresses and warm sitz baths. Larger hematomas involving nearby structures may need operative intervention. Additionally, any evidence of necrosis or rapid expansion should be referred immediately for surgical correction. Superficial vulvar lacerations less than 3 cm typically do not require suturing and are treated with topical antibiotic ointment and covered with gauze. Indications for surgical repair with a specialist include lacerations greater than 3 cm, lacerations through or above the hymen, deep lacerations, bleeding of an unclear source, and penetrating injuries. Patients should urinate before discharge to rule out urethral injury. Caretakers should be advised to use sitz baths and gentle hygiene at home. Although most straddle injuries have good outcomes, complications can include urethral strictures and incontinence if injuries are not recognized.[13]

Bartholin Cyst Abscess

Bartholin glands (also known as the greater vestibular glands) are part of a female patient's normal anatomy. They are located at the posterior vulva in the vestibule and secrete mucus for the lubrication of the vulva and vagina. The glands are approximately 0.5 cm in size in adolescents/adults and drain lubricating mucus in a 2.5 cm long duct. Cysts and abscesses at the site of the glands may form when glands become obstructed. The greatest incidence is during the perimenopausal period but obstruction may occur at any age. The most common bacterial culprit is *Escherichia coli* but polymicrobial infections with *Staphylococcus aureus*, and other enteric bacteria are also common. STIs such as *Chlamydia trachomatis* or *Neisseria gonorrhoeae* may also less commonly cause abscesses. Cysts and abscesses typically occur posteriorly at the 5 o'clock and 7 o'clock position of the vulva, adjacent to the vaginal opening.

Table 2
Recommended first-line treatment of common sexually transmitted infections as per the Centers for Disease Control and Prevention 2021 treatment guidelines https://www.cdc.gov/std/treatment-guidelines/default.htm [14]

Disease	Treatment
Chlamydial infections (nasopharynx, urogenital, and rectal)	*Infants and children (<45 kg)* *Erythromycin base* or *erythromycin ethylsuccinate PO*: 50 mg/kg/d orally (4 divided doses) daily for 14 d *Children aged under 8 y (≥ 45 kg): Azithromycin* PO:* 1g orally in a single dose *Children aged 8 years and older: Azithromycin* PO:* 1g orally in a single dose or *doxycycline PO*: 100 mg orally 2×/d for 7 d Adolescents: *Doxycycline PO*: 100 mg orally 2×/d for 7 d
Gonococcal infections (nasopharynx, urogenital, and rectal)	*Ceftriaxone IM*: 500 mg IM in a single dose *Children (≤45 kg) with urogenital or rectal disease: Ceftriaxone IV or IM*: 25–50 mg/kg IV or IM, not to exceed 250 mg IM in a single dose
Pelvic inflammatory disease, mild-to-moderate outpatient regimen	*Ceftriaxone IM*: 500 mg IM in a single dose *PLUS doxycycline PO*: 100 mg orally 2×/d for 14 d *PLUS metronidazole PO*: 500 mg orally 2×/d for 14 d
Pelvic inflammatory disease, severe inpatient regimen	*Ceftriaxone IV*: 1 g IV every 24 h *PLUS Doxycycline PO or IV*: 100 mg orally or IV every 12 h *PLUS Metronidazole PO or IV*: 500 mg orally or IV every 12 h or *Cefotetan IV*: 2g by IV every 12 h *PLUS doxycycline PO or IV*: 100 mg orally or IV every 12 h or *Cefoxitin IV*: 2 g IV every 6 h *PLUS doxycycline IV*: 100 mg orally or IV every 12 h
Genital herpes simplex (first clinical episode)	*Acyclovir PO*: 400 mg orally 3×/d for 7–10 d or *Valacyclovir PO*: 1 g orally 2×/d for 7–10 d or *Famciclovir PO*: 250 mg orally 3×/d for 7–10 d
Bacterial vaginosis	*Metronidazole PO*: 500 mg orally 2×/d for 7 d or *Metronidazole gel 0.75%*: One 5 g applicator intravaginally 1×/d for 5 d or *Clindamycin 2% topical cream*: One 5 g applicator intravaginally at bedtime for 7 d
Trichomoniasis	*Metronidazole PO*: 500 mg orally 2×/d for 7 d

* Azithromycin is the recommended treatment in pregnancy.

Differential diagnosis includes labial abscess, perineal abscess, or hernias. Treatment of a small (<3 cm) Bartholin cyst includes supportive treatment with sitz baths, good hygiene, and analgesics. Bartholin abscesses require drainage, which can be performed at the bedside. Antibiotics can be considered in patients with overlying cellulitis, concomitant urinary tract infection, pregnancy, immune compromise, signs of systemic infection, or STIs.

Sexually Transmitted Infections

STIs are extremely common worldwide and affect 1 in 5 people in the United States. There is a wide spectrum of symptoms that require evaluation for STIs. Some patients are asymptomatic and diagnosed on routine screening, whereas others may have symptoms of dysuria, vaginal discharge, inguinal lymphadenopathy, or genital ulcerations. Additionally, generalized systemic symptoms such as fever, joint pain, weight loss, and rash may accompany certain STIs. STI recognition is important, not only because of their prevalence but also because of the significant complications that can develop if untreated such as pelvic inflammatory disease, infertility, tubo-ovarian abscesses, and chronic pelvic pain. STIs can also be a presenting symptom of sexual abuse in a child or adolescent, and thus recognizing this diagnosis is paramount in caring for a child.

Confirming the diagnosis of a sexually transmitted infection begins with a thorough history. Confidential discussions without parents or caregivers in the room facilitate more honest conversations in many adolescents. The CDC advocates for the 5 "P's" of a sexual history, including partners, practices (vaginal, rectal, oral), protection, past history of STIs, and pregnancy intention. In cases of suspected sexual abuse, providers should take care to document exactly what the child says and avoid any leading questions, by either caretakers or providers.

Table 1 describes presenting symptoms of common STIs, and **Table 2** summarizes recommended treatment regimens. Empiric treatment should be considered for patients and patients' partners, especially given the unique challenges in securing follow-up for adolescents who wish to remain confidential from caretakers. Most patients with STIs can be discharged with outpatient follow-up. Indications for admission include concomitant sepsis, tubo-ovarian abscess, or pregnancy. Oral intolerance or certain social circumstances where a patient is unable to comply with outpatient medical management may require inpatient antibiotics. Additionally, any child with suspected sexual abuse mandates further investigation.

Pelvic inflammatory disease is a complication of chlamydia and gonorrhea and remains common in adolescents. Additionally, it may be caused by a variety of other organisms. Patients may present with mild or vague symptoms, including vaginal bleeding, discharge, or dyspareunia with pelvic pain. In sexually active young women with lower abdominal pain of an unknown cause, or with either uterine, adnexal, or cervical motion tenderness, presumptive treatment of pelvic inflammatory disease (PID) should be started. Treatment guidelines can be found in **Table 2**. Because of the difficulty in diagnosis, providers should have a high index of suspicion for PID to prevent future complications such as infertility and ectopic pregnancies.

CLINICS CARE POINTS

- Normal maternal estrogen effects on the neonate include vaginal discharge, vaginal bleeding, and breast buds in the first several weeks of life.
- Prepubertal pediatric patients presenting with gynecologic complaints should have external gynecologic examinations only. If internal examinations are indicated, it should be performed under anesthesia.
- Prepubescent girls commonly develop vulvovaginitis that is typically secondary to poor hygiene and local irritation. *Candida* infection is rare before puberty.
- Straddle injuries are potentially more severe with a penetrating mechanism, which warrants a more extensive evaluation.

- Ovarian torsion is most commonly associated with a mass but prepubescent children may torse a normal ovary to due hypermobile adnexa.
- Doppler ultrasound is incompletely sensitive for the diagnosis of ovarian torsion secondary to dual arterial supply.
- Many inguinal hernias contain the ovary and/or fallopian tube. Torsion must be considered with acute pain at the hernia site.
- Sexually transmitted infections are common in adolescence. Screening and empiric treatment should be frequently offered during emergency department visits.

DISCLOSURE

The authors have nothing to disclose.

REFERENCES

1. Castets S, Nguyen KA, Plaisant F, et al. Reference values for the external genitalia of full-term and pre-term female neonates. Arch Dis Child Fetal Neonatal Ed 2021; 106(1):39–44.
2. Howell JO, Flowers D. Prepubertal Vaginal Bleeding: Etiology, Diagnostic Approach, and Management. Obstet Gynecol Surv 2016;71(4):231–42.
3. Lee KH, Hong JS, Jung HJ, et al. Imperforate Hymen: A Comprehensive Systematic Review. J Clin Med 2019;8(1):56.
4. Rose E, editor. Pediatric emergencies: a practical, clinical guide. Online edition. 2020. New York: Oxford Academic, Available at: https://doi.org/10.1093/med/9780190073879.001.0001. Accessed July 26, 2022.
5. Eyk NV, Allen L, Giesbrecht E, et al. Pediatric vulvovaginal disorders: a diagnostic approach and review of the literature. J Obstet Gynaecol Can 2009;31(9):850–62.
6. Loveless M, Myint O. Vulvovaginitis- presentation of more common problems in pediatric and adolescent gynecology. Best Pract Res Clin Obstet Gynaecol 2018;48:14–27.
7. Mashiach R, Melamed N, Gilad N, et al. Sonographic diagnosis of ovarian torsion: accuracy and predictive factors. J Ultrasound Med 2011;30(9):1205–10.
8. Wilkinson C, Sanderson A. Adnexal torsion – a multimodality imaging review. Clin Radiol 2012;67(5):476–83.
9. Wang JH, Wu DH, Jin H, et al. Predominant etiology of adnexal torsion and ovarian outcome after detorsion in premenarchal girls. Eur J Pediatr Surg 2010; 20(5):298–301.
10. Anders JF, Powell EC. Urgency of evaluation and outcome of acute ovarian torsion in pediatric patients. Arch Pediatr Adolesc Med 2005;159(6):532–5.
11. Tsai J, Lai JY, Lin YH, et al. Characteristics and Risk Factors for Ischemic Ovary Torsion in Children. Children 2022;9(2):206.
12. Merriman TE, Auldist AW. Ovarian torsion in inguinal hernias. Pediatr Surg Int 2000;16(5–6):383–5.
13. O'Brien K, Fei F, Quint E, et al. Non-Obstetric Traumatic Vulvar Hematomas in Premenarchal and Postmenarchal Girls. J Pediatr Adolesc Gynecol 2022. https://doi.org/10.1016/j.jpag.2022.03.006. S1083-3188(22)00185-1.
14. Centers for Disease Control and Prevention. Provider Resources. 2022. Available at: https://www.cdc.gov/std/treatment-guidelines/provider-resources.htm. Accessed 1 July, 2022.

Intimate Partner Violence and Sexual Violence

Benjamin Chan, MD, MPH*, Carolyn Joy Sachs, MD, MPH

KEYWORDS

- Intimate partner violence • Sexual violence • Sexual assault • Teen dating violence

KEY POINTS

- Questions: What are intimate partner violence (IPV) and sexual violence (SV), and how do clinicians effectively identify and help patients suffering from them?
- Findings: IPV and SV are very common and occur in persons from all socioeconomic backgrounds, religious, and cultural groups. Numerous individual, relationship, community, and societal factors all play into both a victim's risk of IPV or SV and a person's likelihood of becoming a perpetrator.
- Meaning: Identifying and optimally caring for persons suffering with IPV and SV requires a preplanned multidisciplinary approach involving clinicians, nurses, community workers, social workers, sexual assault nurse/forensic examiners, and nonclinician mentors.

INTIMATE PARTNER VIOLENCE

Introduction

According to The World Health Organization, intimate partner violence (IPV) refers to behavior by an intimate partner or ex-partner that causes physical, sexual, or psychological harm, including physical aggression, sexual coercion, psychological abuse and controlling behaviors.[1] Intimate partners may be spouses, domestic partners, boyfriends/girlfriends, dating partners, sexual partners, or other romantic type of relationship and can be current or former partners, of the same or opposite sex, and may or may not be cohabitating. IPV can be in the form of acts or threats of physical violence, psychological/emotional aggression, controlling behaviors, or sexual violence (SV) between intimate (or formerly intimate) partners. Physical violence can manifest itself in many different forms but its essence is when one partner attempts to harm another partner using force or other physical means. Psychological aggression is the use of verbal and nonverbal communication to control, threaten, or manipulate another person mentally or emotionally. SV is the act or threat to attempt or complete sexual contact with a person without legal consent. SV and assault will be discussed later in the article in a separate dedicated section.

UCLA Ronald Reagan | Olive View, 924 Westwood Boulevard, Suite 300, Los Angeles, CA 90024, USA
* Corresponding author.
E-mail address: BHChan@mednet.ucla.edu

Emerg Med Clin N Am 41 (2023) 369–380
https://doi.org/10.1016/j.emc.2023.01.007
0733-8627/23/© 2023 Elsevier Inc. All rights reserved.

IPV is common and occurs in all socioeconomic backgrounds, religious, and cultural groups. According to the 2010 National Intimate Partner and Sexual Violence Survey (NISVS) conducted by the Centers for Disease Control and Prevention (CDC), more than 1 in 3 women (35.6%) and more than 1 in 4 men (28.5%) in the United States have experienced rape, physical violence, and/or stalking by an intimate partner in their lifetime. More than 43 million women and 38 million men have experienced psychological aggression by an intimate partner in their lifetime.[2] In the year preceding the survey, approximately 5.9% or 7 million women reported IPV. Furthermore, IPV does not just occur in adults. When IPV occurs in adolescence, it is referred to as teen dating violence (TDV). Another CDC survey, the Youth Risk Behavior Survey in 2019, indicates that 1 in 12 US high school students experienced physical dating violence and 1 in 12 also experienced sexual dating violence among high school students who reported dating in the 12 months before the survey.[3]

Several risk factors have been found to increase the risk of IPV. These can be divided into individual factors, relationship factors, community factors, and societal factors. Some individual risk factors that increase a person's risk for perpetrating an act of IPV against their partner include young age, low level of education, witnessing or experience violence as a child, use of alcohol and drugs, personality disorders, acceptance of violence (feeling that it acceptable to beat their partner), and past history of abusing partners. Although women of all ages may experience IPV, it is most prevalent among women of reproductive age and contributes to gynecologic disorders, pregnancy complications, unintended pregnancy, and sexually transmitted infections (STIs).[4] Relationship risk factors include conflict or dissatisfaction in the relationship, economic stress, witnessing violence between parents as a child, and disparity in educational attainment. Finally, the community and societal factors that contribute to increasing IPV are gender-inequitable social norms, traditional gender norms, lack of women's civil rights, weak community sanctions against IPV (eg, unwillingness of neighbors to intervene when they witness violence), poverty, broad social acceptance of violence as a way to resolve conflict, and armed conflict and high levels of general violence in society.[5,6] In TDV, female students and students who identified as lesbian, gay, bisexual, transgender, or queer, or those who were unsure of their gender identity experienced higher rates of both physical and sexual dating violence compared with their counterparts.[7] Contrarily, protective factors against IPV perpetration include strong social support networks, a stable positive relationship, access to stable safe housing, access to medical and mental health services, and access to financial help.[6]

IPV represents a significant and challenging public health issue carrying many individual and societal costs. These can include physical injury, other negative health outcomes, and even death. More than 1 in 3 female and 1 in 9 male IPV survivors suffer physical injury. Other negative health consequences include physical and mental conditions that can affect every system of the body. IPV victims are at increased risk for substance use disorders, high-risk sexual contact, depression, and posttraumatic stress disorder. US crime reports suggest that around 20% of homicide victims are killed by an intimate partner. Moreover, more than 50% of female homicide victims in America are perpetrated by current or former male intimate partners. The financial cost of IPV on society is estimated to be US$3.6 trillion with the cost per victim being US$103,767 for women and US$23,414 for men during their lifetime. This sum total includes costs incurred by medical services related to IPV, lost productivity, and criminal justice costs.[8]

TDV is an adverse childhood experience, which may induce severe consequences in developing teenagers. Similar to their adult counterparts, teens are prone to experience increased depression, suicidal thoughts, anxiety, and increased substance use behaviors. They can also exhibit antisocial behaviors such as lying, theft, and bullying. TDV increases the risk of perpetuating the cycle of IPV and SV throughout life as well.[3]

Terminology

In this article, we often use the term "victim" to describe patients suffering from IPV and/or SV. However, when speaking with patients, it is best to avoid the term "victim" and replace it with the more empowering moniker of "survivor."

Identification

As medical practitioners, our goal will be focused on the secondary and tertiary prevention of IPV. This often involves a multidisciplinary approach to identification, treatment, and referral. Secondary prevention is defined as screening to identify diseases in the earliest stages, before the onset of signs and symptoms (ie, mammography and regular blood pressure testing). The management of a disease after diagnosis in order to slow or stop the progression of a disease is tertiary prevention (ie, chemotherapy, rehabilitation, and screening for complications). However, primary prevention is the act of intervening before health effects through efforts such as vaccination, risky behavior modification, or banning harmful substances.[9] Primary prevention of IPV naturally targets perpetrators and involves changing social norms and providing serious consequences for offenders. Clinicians play an important role in primary, secondary, and tertiary prevention and treatment of IPV.

The American Congress of Obstetricians and Gynecologists (ACOG), along with the United States Department of Health and Human Services, and the Institute of Medicine recommend that IPV screening and counseling be part of preventive care and obstetric care. In addition to screening, providers should offer ongoing support and review available prevention and referral options. Many times, the barrier for clinicians include time constraints, discomfort with the topic, fear of offending the patient or partner, the need for privacy, perceived lack of power to change the problem, and a misconception regarding the population's risk of exposure to IPV.[4]

There are multiple screening tools that can be used to identify patients who are at risk for IPV. The tools with the highest sensitivity and specificity evaluated by the US Preventive Services Task Force were the HITS (hurt, insult, threaten, scream)—refer to **Box 1**, OVAT (Ongoing Violence Assessment Tool), STaT (slapped, threaten, and throw), HARK (humiliation, afraid, rape, kick), CTQ–SF (Modified Childhood Trauma Questionnaire–Short Form), and the WAST (Woman Abuse Screen Tool).[10] These screening questionnaires can either be self-administered or delivered by a clinician in an interview format. Given that patient disclosure may not occur at the first screening attempt, it is important to have regular screenings. For example, during a patient's obstetrics visit, screening should occur at the first prenatal visit, at least once per trimester, and at the postpartum checkup.

Before broaching the subject, it is important to set up the environment to be conducive to obtaining accurate answers. One vital component for success is ensuring patient privacy. This includes interviewing the patient in private without their partner or any other relative or friend in the room. More importantly, questioning a patient about IPV when with an abusive partner in the room can lead to further acts of IPV and worsen the victim's situation. It may also help to preface the encounter with reassurances of confidentiality during the interview with the caveats of mandatory reporting situations. Many times, patients do not recognize themselves as victims or do not want to label themselves this way. Open-ended questioning allows for the patient to

---

Box 1
HITS[11]

Hurt, insult, threaten, and scream

How often does your partner physically Hurt you?

How often does your partner Insult or talk down to you?

How often does your partner Threaten you with physical harm?

How often does you partner Scream or curse at you?

Scoring procedures: Each question is answered on a 5-point scale:

1 = never, 2 = rarely, 3 = sometimes, 4 = fairly often, 5 = frequently

The scores range from 4 to a maximum of 20. For female patients, a HITS cutoff score of 10 or greater was used to classify participants as victimized; for male patients, a HITS cutoff score of 11 or greater was used to classify participants as victimized.

---

tell the provider what is worrying them and gives them space to discuss their situation. Having a nonjudgmental and nonthreatening approach also facilitates successful disclosure. It can be difficult to admit to a new provider that they are in a vulnerable situation. Again, disclosure may not occur during the patient's initial screening, and having a good patient rapport by creating and maintaining trusting relationships is key to disclosure of sensitive information. Another role of physicians is to educate the patient. Oftentimes, this is difficult in the office or emergency department (ED) setting. If IPV is not divulged, a disclosure should not be forced. More importantly, the patient should be offered support, community resources, and the opportunity to return for assistance. By providing the patient with education and resources, they can still receive the useful information and use it when it is most appropriate for them. Moreover, discussing the aspects of safe and healthy relationships serves as primary prevention and may prevent serious abuse from occurring later on by helping the patient identify red flags that may precede acts of IPV.

Clinical Features

There is no specific pattern of injury that has a good predictive value for IPV. Therefore, clinicians must always maintain a suspicion for IPV, especially in vulnerable populations. Many suffering from IPV present to the clinic or the ED with various complaints including gynecologic complaints, uncontrolled medical illnesses, mental health or substance use issues, or chronic pain. Missed medical appointments, medication noncompliance, and delays in seeking medical treatment are some findings that may increase suspicion for IPV. In these situations, the perpetrator may be preventing the patient from accessing care. Additional clues for IPV are examination findings that are not consistent with the history, multiple injuries in the past, patients stating that they are accident-prone, or a vague or changing history. These should prompt the clinician to probe deeper and more specifically regarding IPV.

Some patterns of injury that may be seen in IPV include facial or neck trauma, genitourinary trauma, bilateral trauma (trauma to both extremities), central location of trauma (ie, trunk, breasts), defensive injuries (ulnar aspect of forearm, injury to the axilla), injuries in different stages of healing, and patterned injuries (cigarette burns). Perpetrators often use strangulation as a means to intimidate and injure victims, and subconjunctival hemorrhages are frequently found during the physical examination hours to days after such injury (**Fig. 1**). Clinicians should document location, size,

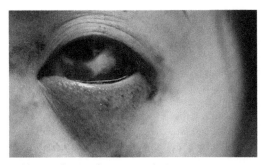

Fig. 1. Subconjunctival hemorrhage after strangulation.

swelling, pain, stages of healing, and patterns of injury. This can be facilitated by uploading pictures of the injuries into the electronic medical record with the patient's consent. Many IPV victims present with gynecologic and obstetric complaints as well (**Fig. 2**). These include frequent STIs, repeated encounters for emergency contraception or termination of pregnancy, or pregnancy-related complications.

Management

Management of a patient that discloses IPV includes treatment of injuries, emotional support, and referral to additional services. Diagnostic testing for injuries or conditions related to IPV follow general medical, trauma, or psychiatric guidelines.

After disclosure, give supportive statements to the patient. These statements can make the patient feel more at ease, let them know that they are working together with you as a team, and can lead to better adherence to recommendations. Recognize the importance of this moment and honor their vulnerability in disclosing. For example, you can say, "Thank you for sharing this with me. I know it takes a lot of courage." The patient's choice to disclose means that they have a great deal of respect and trust for the clinician. Statements such as, "You are not the only one who has suffered this kind of abuse. IPV is a common problem," affirm acknowledge the patient's experiences. An open-ended follow-up can be as simple as, "How can I best support you right now?" Afterwards, ask permission to involve social workers or other patient advocates. Assess the situation for safety and danger concerns. Some states and local governments mandate reporting of certain injuries or acts to law enforcement or other state organizations and providers need to know the local legislation germane to their

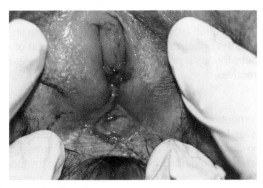

Fig. 2. Injury to the posterior fourchette.

practice area. Finally, make a plan for follow-up with the patient. Reinforce that IPV is a medical condition and normalize that the patient can follow up for further assistance.

A 20-question danger assessment tool, refer to **Box 2**, was developed by Dr Jacquelyn Campbell at Johns Hopkins in 1986 and subsequently validated in a study of IPV-related homicides across 11 cities. The tool identifies factors that often correlated with homicide or attempted homicide in the setting of IPV.

The tool was designed to be used as the basis for discussion with battered women to identify their danger of homicide and to assist in the decision-making process for their situation.[11] After the assessment is completed, the results should be shared with the patient along with consultation of a social worker and/or an IPV advocate to facilitate safety planning and the desired course of action on discharge.

Once clinicians have identified victims of IPV, they can connect patients to multidisciplinary interventions that have been shown to improved outcomes for the patients. Randomized control trials support these interventions that include counseling, home visits, and mentoring support. Counseling includes information on community resources and safety behaviors. Home visits may include parenting support, education on problem-solving strategies, and emotional support. These interventions may be provided by clinicians, nurses, community workers, social workers, or nonclinician mentors.[10]

Referral services can also help with the risk assessment of acute danger to the patient or their dependents, provide methods to increase safety, and determine readiness to separate from the perpetrator. These services should include intervention and referral resources (including safe housing). Legal resources may also be needed in the setting of patients trying to separate from their perpetrator for assistance with custody, orders for protection, and criminal charges.

One systematic review that evaluated the benefits of IPV interventions in primary health settings found that most interventions resulted in reducing violence, promoting safety behaviors, improving physical or emotional health, and/or use of IPV community-based resources. The study concluded that most studies examined demonstrated benefits to patients after primary care IPV interventions, with IPV and/or community referrals being the most commonly improved outcome. Additionally, it noted that successful interventions generally focused on self-efficacy and empowerment, access to IPV resources, and included brief nonphysician interventions and collaborative multidisciplinary care teams.[12]

Involvement of Law Enforcement Agencies

The decision to involve law enforcement agencies should generally be made by the patient unless the situation involves mandatory reporting laws. Victims of aggravated assault or violent crimes, injuries involving firearms or other deadly weapons, and suspected danger to children often legally require reporting. Consulting law enforcement may promptly enhance the patient's safety by immediate arrest or restraining orders. However, if the perpetrator has a prior criminal record, they are less likely to abide by law enforcement directives.

Documentation

Medical record documentation can help future health-care providers and other supportive services deliver high-quality care. Furthermore, it can be used in legal proceedings to assist in obtaining child custody, restraining orders, or victims seeking legal recourse. Clinicians should describe the injuries, noting the location, dimensions, and type of injury. The relationship of the perpetrator to the patient should be documented as well. When documenting, patient statements should be placed in quotation

---

Box 2
Danger assessment[11]

Several risk factors have been associated with homicides (murders) of both batterers and battered women in research conducted after the murders have taken place. We cannot predict what will happen in your case but we would like you to be aware of the danger of homicide in situations of severe battering and for you to see how many of the risk factors apply to your situation.

On the calendar, please mark the approximate dates during the past year when you were beaten by your husband or partner.

Write on that date how long each incident lasted in approximate hours and rate the incident according to the following scale:
1. Slapping, pushing; no injuries and/or lasting pain
2. Punching, kicking; bruises, cuts, and/or continuing pain
3. Beating up"; severe contusions, burns, broken bones
4. Threat to use weapon; head injury, internal injury, permanent injury
5. Use of weapon; wounds from weapon

(If any of the descriptions for the higher number apply, use the higher number.)

Answer these questions Yes or No. The "he" in the questions refers to your husband, partner, ex-husband, or whoever is currently physically hurting you.
1. Has the physical violence increased in frequency during the past year?
2. Has the physical violence increased in severity during the past year and/or has a weapon or threat from a weapon ever been used?
3. Does he ever try to choke you?
4. Is there a gun in the house?
5. Has he ever forced you to have sex when you did not wish to do so?
6. Does he use drugs? By drugs, I mean "uppers" or amphetamines, speed, angel dust, cocaine, "crack," street drugs, or mixtures.
7. Does he threaten to kill you and/or do you think he is capable of killing you?
8. Is he drunk every day or almost every day? (In terms of quantity of alcohol.)
9. Does he control most or all of your daily activities? For instance: does he tell you who you can be friends with, how much money you can take with you shopping, or when you can take the car? (If he tries but you do not let him, check here: ____)
10. Have you ever been beaten by him while you were pregnant? (If you have never been pregnant by him, check here: ____
11. Is he violently and constantly jealous of you? (For instance, does he say "If I cannot have you, no one can.")
12. Have you ever threatened or tried to commit suicide?
13. Has he ever threatened or tried to commit suicide?
14. Is he violent toward your children?
15. Is he violent outside of the home?

____ Total "Yes" Answers

---

marks or preceded with "patient states." If the electronic medical record allows for photographic media to be uploaded into the patient's chart, then the injuries should be digitally photographed and placed in the chart with the patient's consent. In order to provide adequate context for the injury, we recommend uploading at least 4 photographs of each injury. One should be from a long distance away and include the patient's face for identification; one should be from a medium range; and the last 2 should be at a close range with one including a ruler for scale and one without a ruler. These images ideally can be photographed by law enforcement or a forensic specialist. If the patient declines digital photography, they should be encouraged to document their injuries with their own photography to keep a record as these have successfully been used in legal proceedings. Whenever consultations are obtained, whether by referral agencies, social work, IPV advocates, or law enforcement, they should be documented in the medical record as well. Finally, IPV or suspected IPV should be documented in the medical chart for possible use in legal proceedings.

SEXUAL ASSAULT/VIOLENCE
Introduction

Sexual assault/violence is defined as a sexual act that is attempted or committed by another person without freely given consent of the victim or against someone who is unable to consent or refuse. It includes a spectrum of threats or acts including nonconsensual completed or attempted penetration of the vagina, anus, or mouth, nonconsensual intentional touching of a sexual nature, or nonconsensual noncontact acts of a sexual nature such as voyeurism and verbal or behavioral sexual harassment. Although SV perpetrators are more likely to be someone known to the victim,[20] SV can be experienced or perpetrated by anyone. Approximately half of SV patients name an intimate or formerly intimate partner as their perpetrator. SV affects every community and affects people of all ages, genders, and sexual orientations.

Consent is the act of obtaining approval via words or overt actions by a person who is both legally and functionally competent to give informed approval. Examples of situations in which consent cannot be given include underage victims, illness, mental or physical disability, intoxication to the point of incapacitation through voluntary or involuntary use of alcohol or drugs, or being asleep or unconscious. Sometimes encounters where one party is unable to refuse can occur as well. This can happen when disagreement is precluded by misuse of authority or intimidation through the threat of physical violence or possession of guns and/or other weapons.

According to the NISVS, 1 out of 5 women and nearly 1 in 59 men in the United States have experienced an attempted or completed rape in their lifetime. Additionally, an estimated 12.5% of women and 5.8% of men reported sexual coercion. Nearly one-third of women (32.1%) and nearly 1 in 8 men (13.3%) experienced some type of noncontact unwanted sexual experience in their lifetime.[20] However, given the sensitive nature of SV, it is likely that these statistics underreport the true prevalence.

Clinical Features and Medical Consequences

Many traumatic injuries occur in the setting of sexual assault. These can range from minor trauma such as abrasions and ecchymosis to severe such as fractures, urogenital trauma requiring surgery, head trauma, and even in adult female SV victims, the risk of injury increases if the perpetrator is a current or former intimate partner, the encounter occurred in the victim or perpetrator's home, the perpetrator threatens harm to the victim or another, the perpetrator is intoxicated, the rape is completed, or a weapon is used during the assault.[15]

Among women aged 12 to 45 years, the national sexual assault-related pregnancy rate is approximately 5% per rape or around 32,000 pregnancies per year.[13] These rates are particularly high in adolescent survivors because of their higher fertility rates and lower rates of contraceptive use.

Many female survivors of sexual assault may present with chronic pelvic pain, dysmenorrhea, and sexual dysfunction more often compared with those without a history of SV. They may also present with more generalized complaints such as diminished levels of social function, decreased quality of life, increases in various self-reported physical symptoms. Clinicians should recognize and be able to manage the short-term and long-term complications associated with SV including unintended pregnancy, infections, and mental health conditions.

Screening

ACOG recommends that women's health-care providers screen all women for a history of sexual assault, with special care to patients who report pelvic pain, sexual dysfunction, or dysmenorrhea.[14] One validated screening tool for SV is the SAVE screening tool. This tool is a 4-part recommendation that consists of screening all patients for SV, asking direct questions in a nonjudgmental way; validating the patient; and evaluating, educating, and referring.[11]

Examination

If SV survivors communicate beforehand to a physician's office, clinic, or ED, they should be encouraged to go to a medical facility immediately and instructed to refrain from changing clothes, urinating, defecating, cleaning the fingernails, washing out the mouth, bathing, smoking, eating, or drinking. Many jurisdictions use a 72-hour time limit for the collection of evidence in a SV case but others extend that deadline to 7 days. Utmost care must be taken in the SV scenarios because improper evidence collection including incorrect handling of samples or disruptions in the chain of custody can impede legal prosecution of the perpetrator. This is also a very sensitive examination in a vulnerable time period for the patient. Therefore, many hospitals have implemented specialized programs to provide acute medical care and forensic examinations for SV survivors. These programs use Sexual Assault Nurse Examiners (SANEs) or Sexual Assault Forensic Examiners (SAFEs) who have special education and clinical preparation for SV survivors and are well equipped to perform high-quality medical forensic examinations. When a clinician with limited experience is called to perform a sexual assault examination, they should request assistance from the aforementioned trained hospital personnel to ensure that the evidence is gathered appropriately. If no help is available at the facility, then providers can contact the SAFE Technical Assistance program at https://www.safeta.org for clinical guidance and technical assistance.[16]

Management

After the survivor's medical, physical, and legal needs have been addressed, the topic of probability of infection or pregnancy should be discussed. The most common STIs in SV survivors are *Neisseria gonorrheae*, *Chlamydia trachomatis*, and trichomonas infections. The CDC recommends testing and empiric antibiotic treatment of STIs as well as testing for other relevant infections such as human immunodeficiency virus (HIV), hepatitis B virus (HBV), and syphilis. Vaccination for HBV and human papillomavirus is also recommended, as indicated. The recommended antimicrobial regimen for male sexual assault survivors is 500 mg intramuscular ceftriaxone in a single dose (for patients weighing more than 150 kg, 1 gm ceftriaxone should be administered) along with doxycycline 100 mg 2 times a day for 7 days orally. For female sexual assault survivors, the aforementioned regimen is recommended in addition to metronidazole 500 mg twice a day for 7 days. A discussion regarding HIV postexposure prophylaxis (PEP) should be performed with the goal of starting treatment as soon as possible less than 72 hours of exposure. If PEP is started, clinicians should obtain serum creatinine, aspartate aminotransferase (AST), and alanine aminotransferase (ALT) to establish the patient's baseline levels. The patient should be prescribed a starter pack (3–7 days' worth of medications) with a prescription for the rest of the 28 days.[17]

Emergency contraception should be offered to all women of childbearing age. In June of 2022, rape-related pregnancy became an urgent and very dangerous physical and mental health issue for sexual assault survivors in several US states where termination of a pregnancy due to this SV felony act was removed as a treatment option. It is

---

Box 3
Additional resources

- Rape, Abuse, and Incest National Network's (RAINN) National Sexual Assault Hotline
  ○ Call 800.656.HOPE (4673) to be connected with a trained staff member from a sexual assault service provider in your area.
- RAINN National Sexual Assault Online Hotline
  ○ Visit online.rainn.org to chat one-on-one with a trained RAINN support specialist, any time 24/7.
- National Sexual Violence Resource Center
- PreventConnectexternal icon
- Violence Against Women
  ○ Call the OWH HELPLINE: *1-800-994-9662*

---

imperative for practitioners treating sexual assault survivors to choose the most effective emergency contraception available including the copper IUD (**Box 3**)[18,19] and to preemptively provide effective contraception for all patients of childbearing age not actively trying to become pregnant. Levonorgestrel (1.5 mg), known commercially as "Plan B One-Step," has proven exceedingly safe and is currently available in the United States without a prescription. It is effective for up to 5 days after intercourse and has not been associated with teratogenicity if the patient becomes pregnant from the rape or other intercourse in the preceding 7 days. Other forms of emergency contraception include the oral medication ulipristal (prescription only) and the copper IUD, which is effective any time before implantation and more effective in patients with a BMI greater than 30.[19]

Follow-up

Often, other health-care providers, such as the SANE and SAFE providers, should be consulted to provide immediate treatment and intervention for the patient. They can also facilitate counseling and follow-up. Other helpful services include social workers and personnel trained to respond to rape-trauma victims. Further resources can be found on the CDC's website at https://www.cdc.gov/violenceprevention/sexualviolence/resources.html.[20] An SV survivor most likely will not recall all of the information provided during an office or ED visit because of the emotions that they are undergoing during the encounter. Therefore, it is helpful to provide explicit written instructions and follow-up plans in writing. A visit for clinical and psychologic follow-up within 1 to 2 weeks should generally take place with further encounters scheduled as needed based on results and evaluations.

Summary: Provider's role interfacing with patients suffering from partner or SV.

Identification: ask

- Patients may self-present or be transported by prehospital care with trauma.
- Known to be IPV or from SV. Others may require additional queries to uncover the issue.
- Directed screening involves questioning those with risk factors (Sequela described below) about IPV and SV.
- Routine screening involves asking all patients about IPV and SV.

Treatment

- Medical for injuries and forensic sexual assault examination if desired by SV patients.

- Support: This most often involves giving support and information and does not mean a victimized patient will always leave her/his perpetrator or that a survivor of SV will choose a forensic examination and prosecution. Physicians must accept that intervention may be an ongoing process and not easily resolved in one encounter.
- Danger assessment (often with social work and/or advocate or with MyPlan App)

Documentation

- Medical record
- Reporting forms if applicable
- Photography if applicable and available

Referral: will be patient

- Minimum: IPV/SV community resources
- Hospital social work
- IPV/SV community/legal advocate
- Arranging a forensic sexual assault examination by a local forensic examiner program if applicable
- Law enforcement (depending on patient preference and/or mandatory reporting)
  - Reporting may be mandated by state law in certain cases
    - Patients with certain injuries/weapon use
    - When children are involved (to child protective services)
    - When the victim is also a dependent adult or elder (to adult protective services)
    - SV survivors are entitled to a forensic examination without the need to report to talk with law enforcement
    - Mandated reporting supersedes the patient's right to privacy under the Health Insurance Portability and Accountability Act (HIPAA)

CLINICS CARE POINTS

- When questioning patients about IPV make sure the patient is alone.
- Treatment of IPV involves identification, treatment of any injuries, providing kind supportive words, documentation, and referral.
- Referral in IPV involves social work, IPV advocates, and possibly law enforcement.
- All patients presenting after sexual assault should be offered a forensic examination and advocate support.
- Providers must know the local protocol to involve a sexual assault examiner quickly when treating patients reporting sexual assault.

FINANCIAL DISCLOSURE

The authors have no relevant financial interest in this book article.

REFERENCES

1. Available at: https://www.who.int/news-room/fact-sheets/detail/violence-against-women. Accessed June 28, 2022.
2. Available at: https://www.cdc.gov/violenceprevention/pdf/NISVS_Report2010-a.pdf. Accessed June 29, 2022.

3. Available at: https://www.cdc.gov/healthyyouth/data/yrbs/pdf/trendsreport.pdf. Accessed June 28, 2022.
4. Available at: https://www.acog.org/clinical/clinical-guidance/committee-opinion/articles/2012/02/intimate-partner-violence. Accessed June 28, 2022.
5. Available at: https://apps.who.int/iris/bitstream/handle/10665/77432/WHO_RHR_12.36_eng.pdf. Accessed June 28, 2022.
6. Available at: https://www.cdc.gov/violenceprevention/intimatepartnerviolence/riskprotectivefactors.html. Accessed June 28, 2022.
7. Available at: https://www.cdc.gov/violenceprevention/intimatepartnerviolence/teendatingviolence/fastfact.html. Accessed June 28, 2022.
8. Available at: https://www.cdc.gov/violenceprevention/intimatepartnerviolence/fastfact.html. Accessed June 28, 2022.
9. Available at: https://www.cdc.gov/pictureofamerica/pdfs/picture_of_america_prevention.pdf. Accessed June 28, 2022.
10. Available at: https://jamanetwork.com/journals/jama/fullarticle/2708121. Accessed June 28, 2022.
11. Available at: https://www.cdc.gov/violenceprevention/pdf/ipv/ipvandsv screening.pdf. Accessed June 28, 2022.
12. Available at: https://pubmed.ncbi.nlm.nih.gov/24439354/. Accessed June 28, 2022.
13. Available at: https://pubmed.ncbi.nlm.nih.gov/8765248/. Accessed June 28, 2022.
14. American College of Obstetricians and Gynecologists. Guidelines for women's health care: a resource manual. 4th edition. Washington, DC: American College of Obstetricians and Gynecologists; 2014.
15. Available at: https://www.ojp.gov/pdffiles1/nij/183781.pdf. Accessed June 29, 2022.
16. Available at: https://www.safeta.org/. Accessed June 29, 2022.
17. Available at: https://www.cdc.gov/std/treatment-guidelines/sexual-assault-adults.htm. Accessed June 29, 2022.
18. Available at: https://files.kff.org/attachment/emergency-contraception-fact-sheet. Accessed June 29, 2022.
19. Available at: https://www.kff.org/womens-health-policy/fact-sheet/emergency-contraception/. Accessed June 29, 2022.
20. Available at: https://www.cdc.gov/violenceprevention/sexualviolence/resources.html. Accessed June 29, 2022.

Emergency Medicine Considerations in the Transgender Patient

Benito Nikolas Pascua, MD[a], Pamela L. Dyne, MD[b],*

KEYWORDS

- Transgender • Gender nonconforming • Hormone Therapy • Top Surgery
- Bottom Surgery

KEY POINTS

- Transgender individuals are one of the most marginalized and disenfranchised populations in the United States.
- It is important to the transgender patient to have the medical justification for asking sensitive questions and performing examinations explained to them.
- Patient comfort may hinge on a successful introduction which will require clinicians to understand basic acceptable terminology, phrases to avoid, and a level of comfort in asking questions related to gender identity, gender expression, and sexual orientation.
- Providing adequate care of trans patients may involve asking about gender affirming surgeries. Clinicians should develop comfort in taking an anatomic inventory, proactively providing medical justification in asking, and stating and ensuring the information are kept confidential.
- Do not place a blind foley in a transgender man with obstructive urinary symptoms. Most likely a suprapubic catheter will need to be placed as a bridge to urethroplasty.

INTRODUCTION

Perhaps one of the most marginalized and disenfranchised populations in the United States, transgender individuals are disproportionately affected by housing insecurity, unemployment, and extreme poverty. 41%, compared with the general population's rate of approximately 2%, have attempted suicide. Transgender individuals are four times more likely to be living with human immunodeficiency virus, and are more likely to have survived physical assault (61%) as well as sexual assault (64%). They are more

---

Dr B.N. Pascua has no financial interests to disclose. Dr P.L. Dyne has no financial interests to disclose.
[a] UCLA Emergency Medicine, 924 Westwood Boulevard, Suite 300, Los Angeles, CA 90095, USA;
[b] Olive View-UCLA Medical Center, UCLA David Geffen School of Medicine, 14445 Olive View Drive, Sylmar, CA 91342, USA
* Corresponding author.
E-mail address: pdyne@dhs.lacounty.gov

Emerg Med Clin N Am 41 (2023) 381–393
https://doi.org/10.1016/j.emc.2023.01.003
0733-8627/23/© 2023 Elsevier Inc. All rights reserved.

emed.theclinics.com

likely to be incarcerated, to abuse alcohol or illicit drugs, and to avoid necessary health care secondary to harassment and discrimination in health care settings.[1] Emergency departments and emergency care providers should be equipped with the knowledge to effectively treat this population. Many transgender patients report lack of practitioner knowledge of how their transgender history could pertain to their chief complaint and report educating emergency care practitioners of these connections. Many experience unwanted examinations and feel alienated when health care professionals fail to explain the medical justification behind certain aspects of history and physical examination.[2] The aim of this article is to be a primer for clinicians on how to successfully interact with and treat transgender patients in the emergency department through mindful communication, understanding their unique medications and surgical histories, and how they inform the evaluation and management of emergency medical conditions and complaints.

TERMINOLOGY

Many patients and practitioners use the terms sex and gender interchangeably, but it is important to transgender patients that they are recognized as distinct. An individual's biological sex, male or female, is assigned at birth depending on external anatomy. On the contrary, gender reflects a specific culture's way of conceptualizing masculinity and femininity–constructed by society. For example, in most parts of the United States, society recognizes two genders, male or female. Meanwhile, for ages, Thailand has recognized a third gender as being neither male nor female even though such individuals' anatomy would readily place them in the male or female sex.[3] Gender identity reflects an individual's specific way they see themselves, internally, along a gender spectrum which may be male, female, aspects of both or neither. Gender expression, however, is the way a person communicates gender to society through characteristics like voice, mannerisms, and apparel.

Sometimes these terms are confused with sexual orientation, which denotes sexual or emotional attractions. Using the terms appropriately, for example, a gay cisgender man is an individual who was assigned male at birth, who identifies as a man and is attracted to men. A heterosexual transgender man is an individual who was assigned female at birth, identifies as a man and is attracted to women.[4] See **Table 1** for further terminology.

KEYS TO A SUCCESSFUL INTRODUCTION

- *Ask for preferred name*—this demonstrates an understanding that transgender patients may not use their legal names.
- *Ask for pronouns and include yours after your name and role*—if it is unclear from the chart, simply say, "Nice to meet you. I'm Dr Pascua and my pronouns are he/his. What shall I call you and what are your pronouns?" And if you misspeak and use the wrong pronouns during their encounter, simply apologize, as this can damage the patient relationship and perceived quality of care.[7]
- *Opt for gender-neutral terms whenever possible*—say parent rather than mother or father; spouse/partner rather than wife or husband; genitals rather than penis or vagina.
- *Ask direct questions about gender identity and sexual orientation*—this demonstrates care providers are comfortable with such terms and the heterogeneity they may reflect.[8,9]

Refer to **Table 2** for terms considered derogatory or that have fallen out of favor.

HORMONE THERAPY
Key Medical Considerations for Emergency Medicine Clinicians

- Estrogens increase the risk of venous thromboembolism (VTE).
- Ethinyl estradiol carries the greatest risk of VTE (largely only taken by patients obtaining hormone therapy from illegitimate sources).
- Transdermal formulations of estrogen carry the least risk of VTE.

Table 1	
Currently acceptable terminology[5] "GLAAD media reference guide–transgender terms"[6] "LGBTQIA + glossary of terms for health care teams" "LGBTQIA + health education center"	
Terminology	**Definition**
Sex assigned at birth	Usually male or female, typically based on perceptions of external genitalia or anatomy, also described as biological sex
Gender	A construct of society used to classify a person along a spectrum of masculine to feminine, most often spoken of in the binary of male or female.
Gender identity	Invisible to others, reflecting a person's internal sense of self in being male, female, a combination of the two, or neither.
Gender expression	The visible external way a person shows their gender to others through mannerisms, voice, pronouns, clothing, and bodily characteristics.
Pronoun	The words a person uses to refer to themselves which may be he/him, she/her, zie/zirs, they/them.
Cisgender	A person whose gender aligns with their sex assigned at birth.
Transman/female to male/transgender Man	A person who was assigned female at birth but whose gender identity is male.
Transwoman/male to female/transgender woman	A person who was assigned male at birth but whose gender identity is female.
Nonbinary/genderqueer	Not a synonym for transgender; describing a person who experiences gender outside the binary categories of male or female.
Transitioning	An expansive term that encompasses an individual's journey to acknowledge, accept, and express their gender identity. Typically used in reference to changes made to affirm their gender socially, legally, and physically.
Hormone therapy	Often used by transgender individuals to match secondary sex characteristics that reflect gender identity or prevent the development of further disparate characteristics.
Gender-affirming surgery	Procedural changes to the body to further align a person with their gender identity. Some individuals may refer to this as sex-reassignment surgery or confirming surgery but these terms have fallen out of favor.
Transsexual	A term that should only be used if a person identifies as such but is occasionally used in medical literature to reflect a person who has transitioned through medical procedures. Not a synonym for transgender.
Intersex	An identity term some use who have differences in sexual development. Such individuals may or may not identify with the transgender community.

- Always continue hormone therapy whenever possible and taper if you must discontinue estrogen therapy to delay vasomotor symptoms.
- Spironolactone can be discontinued abruptly in cases of hyperkalemia and acute kidney injury.
- Antiandrogens may lead to dizziness or orthostatic hypotension.
- Though testosterone increases triglycerides and low-density lipoprotein levels, there is insufficient evidence to suggest that this leads to increased rates of cerebrovascular or cardiovascular disease.
- Testosterone therapy can safely be discontinued abruptly if needed.

An ever-growing number of transgender individuals are seeking hormone therapy and it is important for emergency medicine clinicians to have a working knowledge of typical formulations, and well as intended and adverse effects of estrogens, testosterone and antiandrogens. Use of hormones helps trans individuals' physical appearances more accurately align with their gender identities and is proven to reduce gender dysphoria and other mental health problems.[10] During hospitalization, whenever possible, these medications should be continued even if they are not on the hospital formulary. Use of these medications and understanding of their related effects may help to identify disease-specific risk factors like osteopenia, elevations in triglycerides or even risk for venous thromboembolism[11] (*Standards of Care for the Health of Transsexual, Transgender, and Gender Nonconforming People*). It is important to note that much of the data used to identify medication risks are extrapolated from cisgender studies using similar therapies. It should be recognized that many trans individuals may obtain hormone therapy through illicit means due to fear of treatment costs, insufficient insurance coverage, or fear of stigmatization. There are no known associated risks related to hormone therapy and the development of hormone-related malignancy, though transgender patients should be screened appropriately by their primary care physicians for prolactinomas, breast, endometrial, ovarian, and prostate cancers.[12] Refer to **Table 3** for common formulations and dosage of hormone therapy and general associated adverse effects to consider.

Table 2
Terms to avoid[5] "GLAAD media reference guide–transgender terms"[6] "LGBTQIA + glossary of terms for health care teams" "LGBTQIA + health education center"

Sex Change/preoperative/postoperative	This places emphasis on surgery as an essential component of transitioning, when in reality many may never pursue such endeavors and/or consider their transition "complete" without any medical procedures.
Biologically/genetically male or female	This emphasizes biology over gender identity. Currently, the accepted way of referring to this is assigned female or male at birth (AFAB or AMAB).
Transgendered	Describes transgender as something that happened to a person rather than an element of an individual's identity. For example, one would not describe a person as Asianed.
Tranny	Widely seen as a derogatory term though some transgender people may use this term to refer to themselves.
Transvestite	A derogatory term referring to a person who wears the clothes associated with another sex.
Hermaphrodite	A derogatory term used to refer to intersex individuals
Real name	This emphasizes legal over chosen names.

Estrogens

Available in oral, parenteral, and transdermal forms, the greatest concern for transgender patients receiving these medications is that of VTE.[13] Effects can be quite variable but may include breast growth, reduction in testicle size, decrease in erectile function, and increased body fat.[14] Both formulation and duration have effects on risk with data showing increased risk of VTE in trans women relative to cisgender men and women.[15] As it is particularly thrombogenic, ethinyl estradiol should not be prescribed. However, unfortunately this may be the only hormone therapy available to patients obtaining medications from underground pharmaceutical dealers. Transdermal formulations are rising in favor because of the reduced risk of VTE, which is thought to be secondary to bypass of first-pass hepatic metabolism and associated increase in hepatic protein synthesis such as procoagulant factors.[16] The Padua score is one of the most broadly used VTE risk assessments that incorporate a factor of hormone therapy but not the indication. However, it is unclear if this risk assessment accurately reflects risk in transgender individuals because the sex of participants was stated as male or female exclusively in the risk assessment model that was used to derive the Padua score.[17]

Aside from VTE, there are data extrapolated from studies in cisgender women regarding drug-drug interactions with certain enzyme-inducing antiepileptic medications. Both phenytoin and carbamazepine increase hepatic metabolism of estrogens, and estrogen increases the metabolism of lamotrigine.[18] There are some instances where cessation from hormone therapy is unavoidable, such as new diagnosis of an estrogen-sensitive tumor. In such circumstances, to postpone or lessen vasomotor symptoms such as hot flashes and night sweats, estrogens should be tapered and not abruptly discontinued, though no serious adverse effects from abrupt cessation have been reported.[19]

Antiandrogens

Some transgender women who have not had an orchiectomy may use anti-androgen therapy for complete feminization. Antiandrogens work by preventing the effects of androgenic hormones released from the testes. Spironolactone, a medication that most may be familiar with in the context of treating liver disease, heart failure, or polycystic ovary syndrome, is one of the most common medications used for antiandrogen therapy.[13] At twice to four times the dosage used for other medical indications, the potassium-sparing and antidiuretic properties of this medication should keep clinicians mindful of hyperkalemia and volume status in transwomen taking it. Unlike estrogens, spironolactone can be discontinued abruptly if medically necessary.[14]

For a variety of reasons, 5-alpha reductase inhibitors may also be used by transgender patients. Agents such as finasteride and dutasteride can be a path to partial feminization for patients unable to tolerate spironolactone or who continue to exhibit undesired virilized features after orchiectomy or complete androgen blockade. Used also by transmen, these medications can address androgenic hair loss, but may lead to orthostatic hypotension or cause dizziness.[13] A synthetic progestogen, cyproterone, more commonly used in Canada and the United Kingdom, is also often used for its potent anti-androgen effects. Though not approved for such usage in the United States, it is well tolerated and efficacious. Rare cases exist of severe hepatotoxicity as well as arterial and venous thrombosis.[20]

Pediatric or adolescent patients may use gonadotropin-releasing hormone (GnRH) analogs to suppress puberty or to prevent menstruation in transgender men. Leuprolide Acetate, the most common of these analogs, works by blocking GnRH receptors,

Table 3
Hormone therapy: common formulations, dosages, and associated adverse effects[12,13]

Hormone	Dosing Range	Comment	Adverse Effects
Estrogen			
Estradiol oral/sublingual	2 to 8 mg/day	Doses >2 mg should be BID	Decreased BMD, Linked with Coronary Heart Disease Risk and Thromboembolic Events
Estradiol transdermal	100 to 400 mcg	Frequency is product dependent	Decreased BMD
Estradiol cypionate IM	2 to 5 mg IM q 2 wk	May divide dosage weekly	
Estradiol valerate IM	20 to 40 mg IM q 2 wk	May divide dosage weekly	
Progestagen			
Medroxyproesterone acetate (provera)	5 to 10 mg qhs		Decreased BMD
Micronized progesterone	100 to 200 mg qhs		
Androgen blocker			
Spironolactone	50 to 200 mg bid		Hyperkalemia, volume depletion
Finasteride	5 mg qday		Orthostatic hypotension, hepatotoxicity, thrombosis, Decreased BMD
Dutasteride	0.5 mg qday		
Androgen			
Testosterone cypionate	50 to 100 mg/wk IM/SQ	May double dosage for q 2 wk frequency	Thrombogenic erythrocytosis, may affect BMD
Testosterone enthanate	50 to 100 mg/wk IM/SQ	May double dosage for q 2 wk frequency	
Testosterone topical gel 1%	50 to 100 mg q AM		
Testosterone topical gel 1.62%	40.5 to 103.25 mg q AM		
Testosterone axillary gel 2%	60 to 120 mg q AM		
Testosterone patch	4 to 8 mg q PM		
Testosterone cream	50 to 100 mg	Frequency varies by compounding pharmacy	

Abbreviation: BMD, bone marrow density.

reducing the release of luteinizing and follicle-stimulating hormones. There are no long-term studies of GnRH analog usage in adults, though concern for reductions in bone-mineral density are shared by current expert guidance.[21]

Testosterone

Available in oral, buccal, injectable, implantable, and transdermal forms, the greatest concern of testosterone use in transmen is that of a thrombogenic erythrocytosis.[13] Despite the United States Food and Drug Administration's issuance of a warning against associated potential venous blood clots from erythrocytosis,[22] meta-analysis of testosterone usage in transmen has revealed that there are insufficient data to determine the true risk of VTE in this population.[23] In addition, despite significant increases in triglycerides and low-density lipoprotein levels after initiating testosterone therapy,[23] studies have not revealed increased cerebrovascular or cardiovascular disease among transgender men compared with cismales.[24] In transgender patients on testosterone who have undergone orchiectomy, abrupt cessation, be it during hospitalization, loss of access to medication refills, etc., though physiologically safe, may lead to hot flashes, mood changes, and fatigue.[12]

NONSURGICAL BODY MODIFICATIONS
Key Considerations for Emergency Medicine Clinicians

- Binding may lead to neurologic, cutaneous, or musculoskeletal complaints.
- Advise patients to limit binding to 12 h a day and avoid it when sleeping or when skin breakdown is present.
- Tucking can lead to testicular torsion, genitourinary infections, and infertility.

Binding or Breast Wrapping

Binding is a practice that many transgender men or gender nonconforming individuals choose to reduce dysphoria associated with a feminine-appearing chest and in turn promote mental health. Also called breast wrapping, a wide variety of materials or combinations of them are used to flatten the appearance of the chest. Tight binding with materials such as ACE wraps or Duct tape can restrict respiration, reduce tidal volume, and lead to rib fractures and pressure ulcers. This may lead trans men to present in the ED setting with chest pain, shortness of breath, or other neurologic, cutaneous, or musculoskeletal complaints of the chest.[25] Though discomfort related to binding is common, patients may be reluctant to share these concerns out of fear they will lead to undesired chest examinations or stigmatization. Although one must examine skin carefully for signs of infection if appropriate for the complaint, ED clinicians should initiate conversations related to binding and be prepared to offer medical advice while limiting the need for physical examination of the affected area if it is not indicated.[25] Patients should be advised to limit binding to a maximum of 12 h a day and avoid wearing such materials while sleeping. Skin breakdown, if present, should be a signal to cease breast wrapping and use skin barriers until resolved.

Tucking

Tucking is a practice that alters the visual appearance of the male groin area to hide or minimizing the appearance of external genitalia to a visibly smooth appearance. The practice is used in a variety of circumstances by trans women to reduce dysphoria or even by drag performers who do not identify as trans. The testes are typically pressed into the inguinal canals while the scrotum and penis are placed between the buttocks.[26] Special support underwear called a gaff or different grades of tape may be used to hold the tuck in place. Skin inflammation from nonmedical grade adhesives is common. Research on the physical effects of this practice is extremely limited and much of the available literature reflects collections of anecdotal accounts from physicians who work with trans patients.[27] Manipulation of external genitalia can lead to a variety of complications. Relocation of the testes may result in pain, inflammation, or even torsion. Prolonged tucking and positioning of the urethral meatus near the anus can lead to urinary tract infections, prostatitis, epididymitis, or orchitis. Mechanical stress from pulling may lead to urethral or skin tears. Fertility issues may be experienced as the anatomical location of the testes is typically at temperatures cooler than core but their placement inside the inguinal canal due to tucking places them is at a higher body temperature.[28]

ANATOMIC INVENTORY

Understanding what gender-affirming procedures or surgeries a patient has undergone can be key to providing timely treatment for emergent pathology. This will inform clinicians of risk factors for disease and affect the differential diagnosis for a chief complaint. For example, ovarian torsion may be possible in a transgender man, but this can likely be ruled out if an adequate anatomic inventory reveals a history of total abdominal hysterectomy with bilateral salpingoopherectomy.[29] Refer to **Fig. 1** when considering taking an anatomic inventory.

Tips on Phrasing

- *Start with a normalizing statement*—indicate you understand transitioning looks different for every trans patient. "Some people undergo gender-affirming surgeries..." Remember, gender-affirming surgery may not be in your patient's goals, financial coverage, or maybe precluded due to lack of specialist availability to perform such procedures.[30]
- *Explain why you are asking*—indicate the medical justification behind seeking this information. "... procedures in this area can have specific impacts on your health and might be related to the reason you came in today." If no medical justification in asking is readily apparent, consider if the knowledge is necessary to address the patient's chief complaint.[31]
- *Ensure confidentiality*—otherwise, you may face considerable reluctance in disclosure for fear of inappropriate treatment or discrimination. "Please trust that I am legally obligated to keep this information confidential."[30]

SURGICAL MANIPULATION
Key Considerations for Emergency Medicine Clinicians

- Top surgery complications are more readily recognizable on physical examination and should involve plastic surgery consultation to ensure cosmetic outcomes are optimized.
- Silicone injection complications are treated supportively and guided by symptoms.
- Bottom surgery is highly variable and when evaluating patients with localizing symptoms, there should be careful consideration of fistula or abscess formation.
- Obstructive urinary symptoms in trans men who have had bottom surgery should not be treated with blind foley placement and instead should be considered for suprapubic urinary catheters as a bridge to urethroplasty.

Currently, most widely used guidelines recommend patients wishing to undergo irreversible surgery, like vaginoplasty and phalloplasty, first live in their gender identity and take gender-specific hormones or hormone suppressants for 12 months.[11]

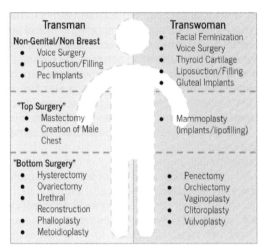

Fig. 1. Gender-affirming procedures.[29]

(*Standards of Care for the Health of Transsexual, Transgender, and Gender Nonconforming People*). Data suggest that approximately 25% of transgender patients have undergone a transition-related surgery.[30] There are three main categories of gender-affirming surgeries: top surgery, bottom surgery, and nongenital/nonbreast surgeries, as described below.

Top Surgery

Top surgery is an umbrella term encompassing all gender-affirming procedures that relate to adjustments in the chest and torso for both transgender men and women. Male chest reconstruction may sometimes include mastectomy or removal of part of breast tissue, and typically involves nipple relocation and strategic contouring to produce a masculine appearance.[32] Such patients may present with postoperative complications such as hematomas, seromas, and nipple complications, Such surgical complications are akin to mastectomy for any indication and should be managed by a plastic surgeon as soon as possible. Transwomen may choose to undergo mammoplasty or breast augmentation, and may develop postprocedural swelling, pain, or deformity. These postoperative complications should be managed by an experienced breast surgeon so as to minimize further complications such as capsular contracture, malpositioning, and asymmetry.[13] Some patients without access to such services through legitimate providers may choose to use illicit silicone injections. This may have catastrophic complications ranging from pain and bleeding to migration, embolization, and localized skin necrosis. Treatment of these complications is largely supportive and guided by symptoms.[13]

Bottom Surgery

Bottom surgery, the second umbrella category, encompasses all procedures related to genital augmentation. Complications are unique and related to the technique used by the surgeon. Vaginoplasty, or creation of a neovagina, has two favored methods: penile inversion or via joining portions of the sigmoid colon to scrotal skin. This includes shortening of the urethra and reconstruction to ensure caudal flow. Postoperative complications may include urinary retention, wound dehiscence, or neovaginal prolapse. Management will include placement and inflation of a large Foley catheter

(20 French or greater), or vaginal packing.[33] Discussion with a urologist who is familiar with the procedure is necessary. Postoperative spotting is typical but one must remain vigilant for potential rectovaginal fistula or perirectal abscesses. As these procedures may result in considerable devascularization between the rectum and neovagina, the postoperative tissue is at risk for necrosis and fistulae may form between the structures.[34] The neovaginal canal requires lifelong dilation and the risk of prolapse increases the further the patient is from their original surgery. Approximately 4% of neovaginas will prolapse, requiring surgical tethering such as sacrocolpopexy or sacrospinous fixation.[35] Yeast-related vaginitis can be treated the same in transwomen as their cisgender counterparts.

Transmen undergoing genital surgery typically choose metoidioplasty or a more complex phalloplasty. In phalloplasty, a variety of techniques using skin and muscle grafts are used to create an increased penile length, usually with the goal of incorporating a prosthesis to aid in penetrative intercourse.[36] As many desire the ability to urinate while standing, phalloplasty typically incorporates a neourethra.[37] Although complication rates have improved from 80% to 40% following phalloplasty, the most common issues continue to develop at the site of urethral anastomosis, namely fistulae or stricture formation.[33] Additional postoperative complications include visible flap loss, groin or pelvic hematomas, and rectal injury along with more common complications of any surgery such as wound infection or breakdown. Out of the acute postop time frame, scarring of the urethra may lead transmen to experience symptoms similar to that of benign prostatic hypertrophy with decreased stream, hesitancy, and retention. Unlike with prostatic hypertrophy, transmen should not have a blind foley placed for these symptoms, with current surgical literature favoring suprapubic catheter placement as a bridge to urethroplasty. Consultation with a urologist familiar with these procedures is strongly recommended.[38] Occasionally, a portion of a pelvic cavity will be unintentionally left intact from an incomplete vulvectomy or colpocleisis. Over time, this region may become a reservoir for urine, manifesting as urinary incontinence of urethrocutaneous fistulae.[13]

Nongenital/Nonbreast

Lastly, nongenital/nonbreast procedures may range from facial feminization or voice surgery to pectoral or gluteal implants. Unlike transgender men whose use of hormone therapy leads to a physical change in vocal folds, transgender women exhibit no change in their voices from the use of antiandrogens or estrogens. Despite extensive voice training, some elect to eliminate the lower sounds of their voice surgically with anterior glottic web formation (functional shortening of the vocal cords) or cricothyroid approximation. Cricothyroid approximation stretches vocal cords by attaching the cricoid cartilage to the thyroid cartilage.[39] Very little data is available relating to the complications of either procedure, but of note, owing to the near obliteration of the cricothyroid membrane, it will likely not be possible to perform an ED cricothyrotomy as an emergent airway intervention on such patients following cricothyroid approximation.

SUMMARY

Transgender patients are at very high risk for poor health outcomes stemming from challenges they may face in accessing medical care for a variety of economic and psychosocial barriers. It is incumbent on emergency care clinicians to have a basic working knowledge of terminology, the effects of hormone therapy, nonsurgical and surgical procedures typically encountered by such patients to provide quality care to transgender patients.

CLINICS CARE POINTS

- It is important for the transgender patient to have the medical justification for asking sensitive questions and performing examinations explained to them.
- Continue hormone therapy whenever possible, even if this means switching to forms that are less prone to venous thromboembolism such as transdermal formulations.
- If estrogen therapy must be discontinued, taper the dosage to reduce vasomotor symptoms.
- Do not place a blind foley on a transgender man with obstructive urinary symptoms. Most likely a suprapubic catheter will need to be placed as a bridge to urethroplasty.
- It may not be possible to perform a cricothyrotomy on a transwoman who has undergone voice surgery as one technique is to close the space between cartilaginous structures, removing the visible cricothyroid membrane.

REFERENCES

1. Grant J., Injustice at every turn: a report of the national transgender discrimination survey. 2011. Transequality.org, National center for transgender equality and the national gary and lesbian task force, Available at: https://transequality.org/sites/default/files/docs/resources/NTDS_Report.pdf. Accessed July 1, 2022.
2. Chisolm-Straker M. Transgender and gender nonconforming in emergency departments: a qualitative report of patient experiences. Transgend Health 2017; 2(1):8–16. Available at: https://pubmed.ncbi.nlm.nih.gov/28861544/.
3. Ocha W. SHORT REPORT: transsexual emergence: gender variant identities in Thailand. Cult Health Sex 2012;14(5/6):563–75. JSTOR, Available at: https://www.jstor.org/stable/23265705.
4. Gold M. "The ABCs of LGBTQIA+." The New York Times, 21 June 2018. Available at: https://www.nytimes.com/2018/06/21/style/lgbtq-gender-language.html. Accessed 12 June 2022.
5. "GLAAD Media Reference Guide - Transgender Terms." GLAAD. Available at: https://www.glaad.org/reference/trans-terms. Accessed 12 June 2022.
6. "LGBTQIA+ Glossary of Terms for Health Care Teams » LGBTQIA+ Health Education Center." National LGBTQIA+ Health Education Center, 3 February 2020. Available at: https://www.lgbtqiahealtheducation.org/publication/lgbtqia-glossary-of-terms-for-health-care-teams/. Accessed 12 June 2022.
7. Lewis MLTK. Trauma in transgender populations: risk, resilience, and clinical care. J Emotional Abuse 2008;8(3):335–54.
8. Haider AH. Emergency department query for patient-centered approaches to sexual orientation and gender identity : the equality study. JAMA Intern Med 2017;177(6):819–28. Available at: https://pubmed.ncbi.nlm.nih.gov/28437523/#:~:text=Nationally%2C%20154%20patients%20(10.3%25),refuse%20to%20provide%20sexual%20orientation.
9. Bjarnadottir RI. Patient perspectives on answering questions about sexual orientation and gender identity: an integrative review. J Clin Nurs 2017;26(13–14): 1814–33. https://pubmed.ncbi.nlm.nih.gov/27706875/#:~:text=A%20majority%20of%20the%20studies,willingness%20to%20disclose%20this%20information.
10. White-Hughto, Jaclyn M. A Systematic Review of the Effects of Hormone Therapy on Psychological Functioning and Quality of Life in Transgender Individuals. Transgender Health 2016;1(1):21–31. https://pubmed.ncbi.nlm.nih.gov/27595141/. Accessed 22 June 2022.

11. Standards of Care for the Health of Transsexual, Transgender, and Gender Nonconforming People. 7, 2012. WPATH, World Professional Association for Transgender Health. Available at: https://www.wpath.org/publications/soc.

12. Rosendale N. Acute Clinical Care for Transgender Patients: A Review. Jama Intern Med 2018;178(11):1535–43. Available at: https://pubmed.ncbi.nlm.nih.gov/30178031/.

13. Deutsch MB, editor. Guidelines for the Primary and Gender-Affirming Care of Transgender and Gender Nonbinary People. 2 ed., 17 June 2016. transcare.ucsf.edu, UCSF, Guidelines for the Primary and Gender-Affirming Care of Transgender and Gender Nonbinary People.

14. Unger CA. Hormone therapy for transgender patients. Transl Androl Urol 2016; 5(6). 877-844. Available at: https://pubmed.ncbi.nlm.nih.gov/28078219/.

15. Getahun D. Cross-sex hormones and acute cardiovascular events in transgender persons: a cohort study. Ann Int Med 2018;169(4):205–13. Available at: https://pubmed.ncbi.nlm.nih.gov/29987313/. Accessed 22 June 2022.

16. Goodman MP. Are all estrogens created equal? A review of oral vs. transdermal therapy. J Womens Health (Larchmt) 2012;21(2):161–9. Available at: https://pubmed.ncbi.nlm.nih.gov/22011208/.

17. Barbar S. A risk assessment model for the identification of hospitalized medical patients at risk for venous thromboembolism: the Padua Prediction Score. J Thromb Haemost 2010;8(11):2450–7. Available at: https://pubmed.ncbi.nlm.nih.gov/20738765/.

18. Johnson E. Caring for transgender patients with epilepsy. Epilepsia 2017;58(10): 1667–72. Available at: https://pubmed.ncbi.nlm.nih.gov/28771690/.

19. Ronit. "Gradual discontinuation of hormone therapy does not prevent the reappearance of climacteric symptoms: a randomized prospective study. Menopause 2006;13(3):370–6. Available at: https://pubmed.ncbi.nlm.nih.gov/16735933/.

20. Bessone F. Cyproterone acetate induces a wide spectrum of acute liver damage including corticosteroid-responsive hepatitis: report of 22 cases. Liver Int 2016; 36(2):302–10. Available at: https://pubmed.ncbi.nlm.nih.gov/26104271/.

21. Hembree WC. Endocrine Treatment of Gender-Dysphoric/Gender-Incongruent Persons: An Endocrine Society Clinical Practice Guideline. J Clin Endocrinol Metab 2017;102(11):3869–903. Available at: https://pubmed.ncbi.nlm.nih.gov/28945902/.

22. LeWine HE. FDA warns about blood clot risk with testosterone products. Harv Health 2014. Available at: https://www.health.harvard.edu/blog/fda-warns-blood-clot-risk-testosterone-products-201406247240. Accessed 23 June 2022.

23. Maraka S. Sex steroids and cardiovascular outcomes in transgender individuals: a systematic review and meta-analysis. J Clin Endocrinol Metab 2017;102(11): 3914–23. Available at: https://pubmed.ncbi.nlm.nih.gov/28945852/.

24. Wierckx K. Prevalence of cardiovascular disease and cancer during cross-sex hormone therapy in a large cohort of trans persons: a case-control study. Eur J Endocrinol 2013;169(4):471–8. Available at: https://pubmed.ncbi.nlm.nih.gov/23904280/.

25. Jarrett BA. Chest binding and care seeking among transmasculine adults: a cross-sectional study. Transgend Health 2018;3(1):170–8. Available at: https://pubmed.ncbi.nlm.nih.gov/30564633/#:~:text=Results%3A%20Of%201273%20participants%2C%2088.9,sought%20care%20related%20to%20binding.

26. Provincial Health Services Authority. "Binding, Packing, Tucking & Padding." Provincial Health Services Authority. Available at: http://www.phsa.ca/transcarebc/care-support/transitioning/bind-pack-tuck-pad. Accessed 22 June 2022.

27. De Roo JM. Addressing tucking in transgender and gender variant patients." Smart Sex Resource, BC Center for Disease Control. 2016. https://smartsexresource.com/health-providers/blog/201610/addressing-tucking-transgender-and-gender-variant-patients. Accessed 22 June 2022.

28. Zevin B. "Testicular and scrotal pain and related complaints." Treatment Guidelines. UCSF Transgender Care Treat Guidlines, 17 June 2016. UCSF transcare, UCSF transgender care. Available at: https://transcare.ucsf.edu/guidelines/testicular-pain. Accessed 22 June 2022.

29. Deutsch MB. Electronic medical records and the transgender patient: recommendations from the World Professional Association for Transgender Health EMR Working Group. J Am Med Inform Assoc 2013;20(4):700–3.

30. James SE. The Report of the 2015 U.S. Transgender Survey. Report. 2016. National Center for Transgender Equality, NCTE, Available at: https://transequality.org/sites/default/files/docs/usts/USTS-Full-Report-Dec17.pdf. Accessed Juy 1, 2022.

31. Chisolm-Straker M. Transgender and gender-nonconforming patients in the emergency department: what physicians know, think, and do. Ann Emerg Med 2018; 71(2):186.

32. Goldstein Z. When Gender Identity Doesn't Equal Sex Recorded at Birth: The Role of the Laboratory in Providing Effective Healthcare to the Transgender Community. Clin Chem 2017;63(8):1342–52. Available at: https://pubmed.ncbi.nlm.nih.gov/28679645/.

33. Santucci RA. Urethral complications after transgender phalloplasty: strategies to treat them and minimize their occurrence. Clin Anat 2018;31(2):187–90. Available at: https://pubmed.ncbi.nlm.nih.gov/29178533/.

34. Davis WD. Emergency care considerations for the transgender patient: complications of gender-affirming treatments. J Emerg Nurs 2021;47(1):33–9. Available at: https://pubmed.ncbi.nlm.nih.gov/33023789/.

35. Buncamper ME. Surgical outcome after penile inversion vaginoplasty: a retrospective study of 475 transgender women. Plast Reconstr Surg 2016;138(5): 999–1007. Available at: https://pubmed.ncbi.nlm.nih.gov/27782992/.

36. Esmonde N. Phalloplasty Flap-Related Complication. Clin Plast Surg 2018;45(3): 415–24. Available at: https://pubmed.ncbi.nlm.nih.gov/29908631/.

37. Morrison SD. Phalloplasty: a review of techniques and outcomes. Plast Reconstr Surg 2016;138(3):594–615. Available at: https://pubmed.ncbi.nlm.nih.gov/27556603/.

38. Nikolavsky D. Urologic sequelae following phalloplasty in transgendered patients. Urol Clin North Am 2017;44(1):113–25. Available at: https://pubmed.ncbi.nlm.nih.gov/27908366/.

39. Seattle Voice Lab. "What to Know About Vocal Feminization." Seattle Voice Lab, 25 November 2021. Available at: https://www.seattlevoicelab.com/what-to-know-about-vocal-feminization-surgery/. Accessed 29 June 2022.

Emergency Gynecologic Considerations in the Older Woman

Nicole Cimino-Fiallos, MD[a], Pamela L. Dyne, MD[b],*

KEYWORDS

- Menopause • Geriatrics • Gynecology • Cancer • Prolapse
- Postmenopausal bleeding • Elder abuse

KEY POINTS

- Pelvic examination is an important step in the diagnosis and treatment of older women with gynecologic complaints and should not be deferred.
- Postmenopausal bleeding is common and affects 20% of older women, but can be a symptom of gynecologic malignancies.
- Pelvic organ prolapse can cause constipation, fecal incontinence, pelvic pain, urinary incontinence, and postmenopausal bleeding.
- Asymptomatic bacteriuria should not be treated with antibiotics in older women, but topical/local estrogen can be used to prevent urinary tract infections.

INTRODUCTION

Older women are the fastest growing segment of the population in the United States[1] and have unique gynecologic emergencies that clinicians must be equipped to manage in the Emergency Department (ED). As women age, they will experience menopause, which is a normal transitional period that affects all body systems. Most women will start to develop symptoms of menopause, which is defined as the absence of menstrual flow for 12 months, between the ages of 40 to 58 years.[2] Although all women will experience menopause as they age, physicians report gaps in knowledge of the expected physiologic changes their patients will develop and may have a limited understanding of the gynecologic emergencies specific to the postmenopausal patient.[3] Differentiating common, but normal symptoms, from

Dr N. Cimino-Fiallos has no financial interests to disclose. Dr P.L. Dyne has no financial interests to disclose.
[a] Emergency Department, Meritus Health, US Acute Care Solutions, 11116 Medical Campus Drive, Hagerstown, MD, USA; [b] Olive View-UCLA Medical Center, UCLA David Geffen School of Medicine, 14445 Olive View Drive, Sylmar, CA 91342, USA
* Corresponding author.
E-mail address: pdyne@dhs.lacounty.gov

Emerg Med Clin N Am 41 (2023) 395–404
https://doi.org/10.1016/j.emc.2023.01.004
0733-8627/23/© 2023 Elsevier Inc. All rights reserved.

emed.theclinics.com

pathologic ailments is a critical skill for emergency practitioners. This article will review the physiology of menopause, common chief complaints among older women, as well as appropriate workup, treatments, and outpatient referrals, which will allow emergency clinicians to feel more confident in their knowledge when caring for this fast-growing demographic.

OVERVIEW OF MENOPAUSE

It is estimated that more than 35 million women in the United States are postmenopausal, with another million women entering menopause each year.[4] Women go through a series of hormonal changes as they mature through menopause. Serum levels of estradiol decrease and levels of follicle-stimulating hormone (FSH) increase. The ovaries begin to produce androstenedione, which is converted by adipose tissue into estrone, which becomes the predominant circulating estrogen.[5] An elevated serum FSH has been identified as a marker for menopause, but it is not sensitive enough to make the diagnosis because levels fluctuate greatly. There is no single laboratory test that diagnoses the onset or completion of menopause, and the diagnosis is made based on the patient's reported symptoms and their age.[6]

As these hormone levels shift, estrogen-responsive organs and pelvic tissues atrophy resulting in friability, devascularization, decreased sensation, and stiffening. Pelvic ligaments weaken and urethral and rectal sphincter tone can decrease. The urogenital tissues experience epithelial thinning and decreased vascularity, resulting in symptoms of vaginal dryness, dyspareunia, and urinary incontinence.

Other body systems are also affected by the changes in this life stage.[6] More than half of all women will experience vasomotor symptoms, frequently referred to as "hot flashes." Approximately 30% to 60% of women will experience sleep disturbances, mood changes, decreased libido, and insomnia (with or without associated night sweats).[6] Cognitive changes, anxiety, depressive symptoms, generalized fatigue, and diffuse joint pain are also common. As women age through menopause, their risk of heart disease, osteoporosis, and diabetes increases. Although systemic symptoms from menopause are common, clinicians should consider their overlap with presentations of other pathologic conditions, such as carcinoid syndrome, hyperthyroidism, and endometrial and ovarian cancers.

Many of the disruptive symptoms of menopause can be managed with pharmacologic treatments. Estrogen therapy can treat vasomotor symptoms, vulvovaginal atrophy, and urogenital symptoms, and can mitigate cardiovascular changes and osteoporosis. Estrogen can be prescribed orally, transdermally, or in a vaginal ring. Using estrogen alone can cause uterine hyperplasia and uterine cancer, therefore estrogen-progestin combination therapies are preferred in patients with a uterus. Progesterone can be taken orally, as a levonorgestrel-releasing intrauterine device, or as a combination estrogen-progesterone patch. Side effects of estrogen therapy include vaginal bleeding, breast tenderness, and nausea. Side effects of progesterone may include mood swings and bloating. Unfortunately, hormone therapy can increase the risk of invasive breast and ovarian cancers, according to data from the Women's Health Initiative (WHI). Hormone replacement therapy (HRT) may also increase the risk of venous thromboembolism.[5] However, decisions about the individual patient's risk of these significant complications of HRT should be weighed against their improvement in quality of life as a result of using HRT.[5] HRT should not be used in patients with a history of breast cancer, endometrial cancer, thromboembolic disease, and coronary artery disease.[5] Patients on HRT presenting to the ED with chest pain or shortness of breath should be evaluated for cardiovascular and thromboembolic events.

HRT should be used at the lowest dose required for the shortest amount of time needed to treat symptoms.

Some physicians may start their patients that are experiencing functional impairment secondary to their menopausal symptoms on selective serotonin reuptake inhibitors (SSRIs), serotonin-norepinephrine reuptake inhibitors (SNRIs), gabapentin, or clonidine.[5] Paroxetine is the only SSRI approved to treat vasomotor symptoms, but venlafaxine is also used off-label. Gabapentin and clonidine have also shown effectiveness in the treatment of vasomotor symptoms. Emergency clinicians should be aware of the indications for these medications for the treatment of menopausal symptoms and the potential adverse effects for older women, specifically, an increased risk of falls caused by SSRIs, somnolence, and ataxia from gabapentin and anti-cholinergic effects, central nervous system depression, and bradycardia from clonidine.[7]

THE PELVIC EXAMINATION IN OLDER WOMEN

When an older woman presents to the ED with a pelvic complaint, a pelvic examination is indicated and should be performed and not deferred. Studies show that deferring pelvic examinations has delayed the diagnosis of pelvic cancers in this population.[1] The patient's symptoms should be discussed before the initiation of this sensitive examination and consider asking the patient for suggestions to make the examination more comfortable. The clinician should inform the patient that each step of the examination will be narrated and that the patient can stop the examination at any time if they are uncomfortable. A frog leg position (where the patient lies on their back, bends their knees with heels together and then abducts the knees) or the left lateral decubitus position (where an assistant holds the right leg up) may be more comfortable than the usually lithotomy position for patients with arthritis or limited range of motion of back or hips.[8] The clinician should perform an external inspection of the patient's urethral opening, vulva, vaginal introitus, and anus. An external examination may be all that is required to address the patient's concerns.

If an internal examination is indicated, generous lubrication should be used as some patients will experience vaginal dryness and stenosis of the vaginal introitus after menopause. The smallest speculum required should be used.[1] A practitioner can offer for the patient to insert the speculum herself. If the physician is inserting the speculum, they should recommend the patient take deep abdominal breaths to relax the pelvic floor muscles. If the frog leg position is used, the speculum handle should be aimed anteriorly, towards the patient's urethral opening.

An internal examination may be more difficult in older women. Topical lidocaine applied to the vaginal introitus may reduce discomfort with the internal examination. If the speculum cannot be inserted without pain, a fecal impaction may be present and compressing the vaginal canal. A rectal examination may reveal a rectocele, rectal prolapse, or fecal impaction.[9] Atrophic vaginitis may make the vaginal tissue more friable and can shorten the vaginal vault, also complicating an internal examination with a speculum.[8] In some patients, such as those with pelvic organ prolapse (POP) and atrophic vaginitis, a speculum examination may not be possible. In these cases, a manual examination with one finger digit should be performed.[8] A manual examination can diagnose retained foreign bodies (such as pessaries), masses, and bleeding.

Patients with cognitive impairment may experience significant anxiety with the pelvic examination. Allowing a support person to stay in the room in addition to having an assistant present during the examination to provide support may improve compliance with the examination. Narrating the examination may also ease anxiety. If available, offering a female examiner may also decrease the patient's anxiety.

POSTMENOPAUSAL BLEEDING AND CANCER

Postmenopausal bleeding is defined as bleeding 6 to 12 months after menopause. 20% of women will experience bleeding after menopause and approximately 10% to 20% of these patients will be diagnosed with a malignancy.[10] The most common cause of postmenopausal bleeding is endometrial atrophy.[11] When evaluating a patient for postmenopausal bleeding, it is important to assess for other potential sources, such as hematuria or hematochezia. Performing a visual inspection of the vulva and a manual examination of the vaginal canal can identify external sources of bleeding like vaginal trauma, polyps, ulcerations, and foreign bodies (eg, retained pessaries). Although uncommon, vulvar and vaginal malignancies do occur and can be apparent on visual inspection. Clinicians should assess for thickened, firm, friable tissues that are asymmetric. Once the clinician has evaluated and excluded these alternative sources of bleeding, endometrial or ovarian malignancy should be considered.

Endometrial cancer typically presents with painless, postmenopausal vaginal bleeding, and a purulent or malodorous discharge may also be reported. It is the most common gynecologic cancer.[12] Risk factors for endometrial cancer include nulliparity, tamoxifen therapy, exogenous estrogen use without progestins, and diabetes.[13] Ovarian tumors can also cause vaginal bleeding in postmenopausal women via hormone secretion. A pelvic examination may discover a palpable ovary, which is always abnormal in an older woman. Patients with new ovarian masses may experience symptoms from mass effect, such as urinary frequency, constipation, pelvic pressure, and bloating. Urinary catheter insertion, pain control, and rectal disimpaction may be required to manage symptoms. Endometrial and ovarian cancers are often difficult to diagnose in early stages and can present with systemic symptoms after metastasis (**Fig. 1**).

Although most workup for a possible malignancy is appropriate for the outpatient setting, a pelvic ultrasound is a reasonable first approach in the ED. Concerning features on pelvic ultrasound may include a complex cyst or a thickened endometrial stripe. Cysts larger than 5 cm are at risk for torsion and gynecology consultation from the ED is indicated. Pelvic ultrasound may be challenging in patients with obesity, fibroids, adenomyosis, or previous uterine surgery.[14] There is a lack of consensus on the cut-off for an abnormal endometrial lining thickness. The American College of Obstetrics and Gynecology recommends further workup when the endometrial lining thickness measures >4 mm. Patients with persistent postmenopausal bleeding should undergo a tissue biopsy even after a normal transvaginal ultrasound, and close outpatient follow-up should be coordinated.[11]

MENOPAUSAL GENITOURINARY SYNDROME

The hormonal changes of menopause can lead to genital dryness, irritation, discomfort, and impaired function of the genitourinary systems. A lack of lubrication and vaginal changes can lead to painful sex and urinary system changes can cause urgency, dysuria, and recurrent urinary tract infections (UTIs).[15] Vulvar and vaginal tissues will change through menopause and patients may experience thinning of the labia and narrowing of the vaginal introitus. On examination, patients may exhibit pale and dry vulvar tissues and the vagina may have a loss of rugae. Patients experiencing vulvovaginitis and atrophy may develop inflammation of the mucosa with erythema and friability.[16] The use of localized estrogen therapy enhances pelvic blood flow and can reverse vaginal atrophy.[5] For women without a history of estrogen-dependent cancers who continue to experience vulvar and vaginal symptoms despite the use of vaginal lubricants and moisturizers, low-dose vaginal estrogen therapy may be appropriate.[17]

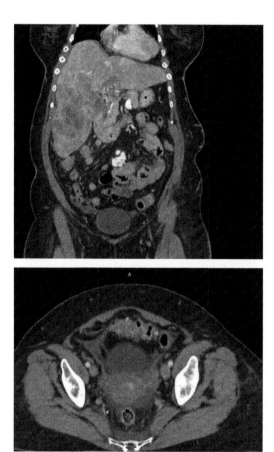

Fig. 1. A 72-year-old woman presented to the ED with intermittent painless vaginal bleeding and abdominal bloating for 3 months. On computed tomographic imaging, the patient was found to have an enlarged uterus suspicious of malignancy and bulky masses in the liver suspicious of metastatic tumors. The patient was also found to have portal vein thrombosis and thrombosis of the inferior vena cava and bilateral iliac veins. (Images courtesy of Dr. Nicole Cimino-Fiallos.)

As women age, the vaginal environment becomes more alkaline and changes to the natural flora make women more susceptible to infections. As the vaginal pH increases, bacterial vaginosis may become more common. Vaginal fungal infections are less common in older women, but the risk of these conditions increases in the setting of diabetes, incontinence, and immunosuppression. When treating vulvovaginal complaints, topical/local therapies are preferred as this patient population is at risk for polypharmacy. Clinicians must also remember that although vulvovaginitis and atrophy are common complaints during menopause and after, other pathologies must be considered. A thick, malodorous discharge can be a symptom of endometrial malignancy. Older adults experience sexually transmitted infections that can cause discharge and pelvic pain. Masses in the vulva are sometimes mistaken for benign Bartholin's cysts, but can actually be malignancies. All pelvic masses should be referred to a specialist to exclude a cancer diagnosis.

GENITOURINARY CONSIDERATIONS

UTIs are common in older women.[18] Urinary incontinence, urinary retention, and menopause all contribute to the increase in UTI frequency in older women due to estrogen withdrawal, weakening of the muscles of the pelvic floor, vascular changes, and alterations in vaginal microbial flora.[19] Vaginal estrogens have shown efficacy in the reduction of UTI frequency. Whether topical cream or a vaginal ring is used, these therapies are safe and do not exhibit the same serious side effects and cancer risks as systemic estrogens. In addition, systemic estrogens have not shown the same benefit of reduction of UTIs as vaginal treatments. Long-term compliance with topical estrogen therapy is the biggest barrier to treatment.

Distinguishing between an infectious process and asymptomatic bacteriuria (ASB) can be challenging in this age group. Recurrent UTIs are more common in postmenopausal women,[20] but more than 20% of women older than 65 and 25% to 50% of women 80 years or older experience bacteriuria.[21] ASB is the presence of 10^5 or more colony-forming units/mL of one or more species of bacteria in the absence of specific genitourinary signs or symptoms attributable to UTI, irrespective of the presence of pyuria.[22] When assessing an older woman for a suspected UTI, it is important to ask about previous UTIs, menopausal status, recent antibiotic use, and sexual history. Sexually transmitted infections can be misdiagnosed as UTIs if a sexual history is not obtained, which may delay appropriate treatment. Older sexually active women with recurrent UTIs should be instructed on early postcoital micturition.[19] Clinicians should avoid treating ASB with antibiotics. Patients with new or worsening urgency, urinary frequency, suprapubic pain, frank hematuria, costovertebral angle tenderness, or new urinary incontinence with a urinalysis consistent with an infection should be treated for a UTI.[23]

PELVIC ORGAN PROLAPSE

POP, including bladder, vagina, and rectum commonly impact older women. A prolapse of the bladder into the anterior vaginal wall is called a cystocele and a prolapse of the rectum into the posterior vaginal wall is called a rectocele. Vaginal childbirth, obesity, chronic constipation, aging, and menopause all weaken the pelvic floor musculature and can lead to POP. A hysterectomy can increase the risk of vaginal prolapse and patients can experience complete eversion of the vagina. Genetic predisposition and connective tissue disorders also contribute to the prevalence of POP.[24]

POP can cause a variety of symptoms. Patients may report pelvic pressure or complain of a bulging mass from the vaginal canal. These symptoms are usually worse in the afternoon/evening after patients have spent the day in the upright position. Patients may experience constipation, incomplete bladder emptying, or urinary or fecal incontinence. The patient may report having to "splint" to initiate urination or defecation, wherein the patient inserts a finger into the vaginal canal to elevate the cystocele or rectocele.[9] In cases of a large prolapse, the patient may notice bleeding and discharge as the vaginal mucosa erodes and becomes ulcerated.

A careful pelvic examination is required to make the proper diagnosis in cases of POP as masses, bleeding and pain can be symptoms of more serious etiologies. Once the diagnosis of a prolapse is established, treatment is based on the severity of the patient's symptoms. In cases of mild prolapse, where symptoms are not disruptive to the patient, observation is reasonable. Patients may participate in pelvic floor muscle strengthening exercises that have shown benefits in mild to moderate prolapse.[24] Pessaries are an option for women that are not surgical candidates or for those that want to pursue nonsurgical treatments. Estrogen cream may improve mucosal quality on exposed vaginal surfaces and decrease ulceration and tissue breakdown. Barrier creams may also be used to protect exposed mucosal surfaces.[9] Emergency practitioners can refer patients to a gynecologist or primary care provider for pessary fitting.[24] Surgical options are available for women who fail conservative treatment options or who desire definitive treatment, although not all older women may be appropriate surgical candidates due to advanced age and comorbidities.

BREAST EMERGENCIES

Although true breast emergencies are infrequent among older women, breast complaints may bring these patients to the ED for evaluation.

Older women may present to the ED for nipple discharge. Practitioners should inquire about laterality (unilateral vs bilateral) and composition (watery, bloody, and purulent). Is the discharge expressed or spontaneous? Although many women will report concerns about possible breast cancer, ductal ectasia and subareolar abscesses are potential non-neoplastic causes of nipple discharge. Ductal ectasia can be a normal part of aging as the subareolar ducts dilate. Spontaneous, unilateral, and clear or bloody discharge is considered pathologic and requires expedient outpatient workup.

Although usually a primary concern of patients, isolated breast pain is not typically the sole presenting symptom of breast cancer. Focal persistent pain is seen in <3% of breast cancers.[25] Breast trauma, Mondor's disease, stretching of Cooper's ligaments, sclerosing adenosis, breast cysts, and diabetic mastopathy can cause breast pain. As systems outside of the breast can also cause mammary pain including acute coronary syndrome, pulmonary embolism, pleurisy, and costochondritis, care must be taken to fully investigate the serious and likely causes of the patient's symptoms.[26]

Nearly half of all breast cancers are in women over the age of 65.[27] Most breast cancers will present with a breast mass. Patients may visit the ED because the discovery of a mass can provoke anxiety. Clinicians should perform a thorough examination including an evaluation of the nipple. Women may develop Paget's disease of the breast, wherein the nipple has a weeping eczematoid lesion. This disease is more common in older women and is typically overlying an inflammatory breast cancer.[28] If a patient presents to the ED with a breast mass or concerning nipple finding, emergency physicians should document the location of the mass by referencing the areola as a clock face and provide symptomatic relief, if indicated (such as protective padding for an inflamed nipple).[25] A painless mass evaluated in the ED is unlikely to be infectious and ultrasound imaging in the ED typically doesn't contribute to making the diagnosis.[29] The patient's mass will need imaging, but this often cannot be accommodated in the ED and should be referred for outpatient follow-up. The clinician should document a differential diagnosis specifically listing cancer and the discussion with the patient that includes the need for follow-up. Written discharge instructions should include details for the follow-up plan and contact information for referral physicians.[26]

SEXUAL ELDER ABUSE

Elder abuse is common and approximately 10% of older adults will experience elder abuse in their lifetimes. Sexual elder abuse is the least common form of elder abuse but can have devastating effects on victims.[30] Elder sexual abuse is defined as non-consenting sexual contact of any kind or as sexual contact with any person not capable of giving consent.[31] Although adult children are the most common perpetrators of physical abuse, intimate partners are more likely to be the perpetrators of sexual violence.[32] Most older women live in the community in homes with their families and not in nursing institutions. Although sexual violence does occur in nursing facilities and can be perpetrated by staff or by other residents, such abuse in facilities is less common than abuse in the community.[33]

Many factors contribute to the underreporting of elder sexual abuse. Often, older women live with and are financially dependent on their abusers. The majority of victims of elder sexual abuse are fully dependent on someone else for their care.[34] The abuser may be the person accompanying the victim to doctor's appointments or ED visits. When considering whether or not to report the abuse, many women are concerned about the ramifications of reporting the mistreatment. Women often find the experience of sexual abuse shameful and are hesitant to report the events. Women may worry that health care professionals won't believe them if they report a sexual assault. Dementia and cognitive dysfunction are also barriers to reporting.

Older women presenting to the ED with vaginal bleeding, pain, recurrent UTIs, vaginal sores, vaginal discharge or anal bleeding or sores may be victims of sexual abuse. The clinician should obtain a detailed history and should use a standardized screening tool to identify possible abuse. Patients should be interviewed independently. Women with any of the aforementioned symptoms should undergo a physical examination to evaluate for signs of trauma and sexually transmitted infections. A forensic examination may be appropriate, and the physician should report suspicions of abuse to the appropriate investigative agency.

DISCUSSION

Understanding the appropriate workup and treatments for common gynecologic concerns of older women is critically important for emergency medicine clinicians. Menopause is a normal part of aging that affects many physiologic systems and causes a variety of symptoms, many of which can bring patients to the ED. By differentiating expected physiologic changes of menopause from pathologic findings, physicians can provide reassurance when appropriate and recommendations for needed follow-up if abnormalities are reported or found. Positioning and careful inspection during a pelvic examination can keep older women comfortable while assessing for abnormal lesions, foreign bodies, trauma, and bleeding. Postmenopausal bleeding always requires a workup to determine a source and to start the process of diagnosing any malignancies. Vaginitis, recurrent UTIs, POP, and breast symptoms can distress patients, prompting them to seek help in the ED. Elder sexual abuse, although uncommon, presents a unique challenge to the ED practitioner. Working knowledge of these categories of complaints and their differential diagnoses are important for all emergency medicine practitioners to provide optimal care for such patients.

CLINICS CARE POINTS

- Pelvic examination is an important step in the diagnosis and treatment of older women with gynecologic complaints and should not be deferred.

- Patients on menopausal hormone therapy, also known as hormone replacement therapy presenting to the Emergency Department with chest pain or shortness of breath should be evaluated for cardiovascular and thromboembolic events.

- Postmenopausal bleeding is common and affects 20% of older women, but can be a symptom of gynecologic malignancy and requires a prompt evaluation.

- Asymptomatic bacteriuria should not be treated with antibiotics in older women, but topical/local estrogen can be used to prevent and primary treatment of recurrent urinary tract infections in select patients.

REFERENCES

1. Lewiss RE, Saul T, Teng J. Review article: gynecological disorders in geriatric emergency medicin. Am J Hosp Palliat Medicine® 2009;26(3):219–27.
2. Kleinman NL, Rohrbacker NJ, Bushmakin AG, et al. Direct and indirect costs of women diagnosed with menopause symptoms. J Occup Environ Med 2013; 55(4):465–70.
3. Jiang X, Sab S, Diamon S, et al. Menopausal medicine clinic: an innovative approach to enhancing the effectiveness of medical education. Menopause 2012;19(10):1092–4.
4. Kvale JN, Kvale JK. Common gynecologic problems after age 75. Postgrad Med 1993;93:263–8, 271-272.
5. Peacock K, Ketvertis KM. Menopause. In: StatPearls [Internet]. Treasure Island (FL): StatPearls Publishing; 2022. Available at: https://www.ncbi.nlm.nih.gov/books/NBK507826/.
6. Karvonen-Gutierrez C, Harlow S. Menopause and Midlife Health changes. In: Halter JB, Ouslander JG, Studenski S, et al, editors. Hazzard's geriatric medicine and gerontology. 7th edition. New York: McGraw-Hill; 2017. p. 591–604.
7. American Geriatrics Society 2015 Beers Criteria Update Expert Panel, et al. American Geriatrics Society 2015 updated beers criteria for potentially inappropriate medication use in older adults. J Am Geriatr Soc 2015;63(11):2227–46.
8. Stiles M, Redmer J, Paddock E, et al. Gynecologic Issues in Geriatric Women. J Women's Health 2012;21(1):4–9.
9. Miller KL, Griebling TL. Gynecologic disorders. In: Halter JB, Ouslander JG, Studenski S, et al, editors. Hazzard's geriatric medicine and gerontology. 7th edition. New York: McGraw-Hill; 2017. p. 629–46.
10. Baekelandt MM, Castiglione M, ESMO Guidelines Working Group. Endometrial carcinoma: ESMO clinical recommendations for diagnosis, treatment and follow-up. Ann Oncol 2009;4:29–31.
11. Braun MM, Overbeek-Wager E, Grumbo RJ. Diagnosis and management of endometrial cancer. Am Fam Physician 2016;93(6):468–74.
12. American Cancer Society. Cancer Facts and Figures 2022. Cancer Facts & Figures 2022| American Cancer Society, 10, July, 2022 https://www.cancer.org/research/cancer-facts-statistics/all-cancer-facts-figures/cancer-facts-figures-2022.html.
13. Committee on Gynecologic Practice of American College Obstetricians and Gynecologists. Practice bulletin - endometrial cancer. Obstet Gynecol 2015;125(4):1006–26.
14. Ragupathy K, Cawley N, Ridout A, et al. Non-assessable endometrium in women with post-menopausal bleeding: to investigate or ignore. Arch Gynecol Obstet 2013;288:375–8.
15. Kagan R, Kellogg-Spadt S, Parish SJ. Practical treatment considerations in the management of genitourinary syndrome of menopause. Drugs & Aging 2019; 36(10):897–908.
16. Shifren JL. Genitourinary Syndrome of Menopause. Clin Obstet Gynecol 2018; 61(3):508–16.

17. Stuenkel CA, Davis SR, Gompel A, et al. Treatment of symptoms of the menopause: an endocrine society clinical practice guideline. J Clin Endocrinol Metab 2015;100(11):3975–4011.

18. Soria N, Khoujah D. Genitourinary emergencies in older adults. Emerg Med Clin North Am 2021;39(2):361–78.

19. Caretto M, Giannani A, Russo E, et al. Preventing urinary tract infections after menopause without antibiotics. Maturitas 2017;99:43–6.

20. Romano JM, Kaye D. UTI in the elderly: common yet atypical. Geriatrics 1981; 36(6):113–5, 120.

21. Walters MD, Karram MM. Urogynecology and reconstructive pelvic surgery. Philidelphia, PA: Mosby Elsevier; 2007.

22. Nicolle LE, Gupta K, Bradley SF, et al. Clinical practice guideline for the management of asymptomatic bacteriuria: 2019 update by the infectious diseases society of America. Clin Infect Dis 2019;68(10):e83–110.

23. Loeb M, Bentley DW, Bradley S, et al. Development of minimum criteria for the initiation of antibiotics in residents of long-term-care facilities: results of a consensus conference. Infect Control Hosp Epidemiol 2001;22(2):120–4.

24. Perkins KE, King MC. Geriatric gynecology. Emerg Med Clin 2012;30(4):1007–19.

25. Freedman RA, Muss HB. Breast disease. In: Halter JB, Ouslander JG, Studenski S, et al, editors. Hazzard's geriatric medicine and gerontology. 7th edition. New York: McGraw-Hill; 2017. p. 1441–7.

26. Lockwood R, Collings JL. In: Breast Disorders" In Adams JG, Barton ED, Collings JL, et al, editors. Emergency medicine clinical essentials. Second edition. Philadelphia: Elsevier; 2013. p. 1114–23.

27. DeSantis CE, Ma J, Gaudet MM, et al. Breast cancer statistics. CA: a Cancer J Clinicians 2019;69(6):438–51.

28. Givens ML, Luszczak M. Breast disorders: a review for emergency physicians. J Emerg Med 2002;22(1):59–65.

29. Roberts JT, Digiacinto W, Nguyen QD. Pitfalls of Breast Evaluation in the Emergency Department. Cureus. 2020 Sep 23;12(9):e10612. doi: 10.7759/cureus.10612. PMID: 33123426; PMCID: PMC7584315.

30. Dong XQ. Elder abuse: systematic review and implications for practice. J Am Geriatr Soc 2015;63(6):1214–38.

31. Tatara T. Suggested state guidelines for gathering and reporting domestic elder abuse statistics for compiling national data. Washington DC: National Aging Resource Center On Elder Abuse (NARCEA); 1990.

32. Brozowski K, Hall DR. Aging and risk: physical and sexual abuse of elders in canada. J Interpersonal Violence 2009;25(7):1183–99.

33. Rosen T, Pillemer K, Lachs M. Resident-to-resident aggression in long-term care facilities: an understudied problem. Aggression Violent Behav 2008;13(2):77–87.

34. Jones H, Powell JL. Old age, vulnerability and sexual violence: implications for knowledge and practice. Int Nurs Rev 2006;53(3):211–6.

Moving?

Make sure your subscription moves with you!

To notify us of your new address, find your **Clinics Account Number** (located on your mailing label above your name), and contact customer service at:

Email: journalscustomerservice-usa@elsevier.com

800-654-2452 (subscribers in the U.S. & Canada)
314-447-8871 (subscribers outside of the U.S. & Canada)

Fax number: 314-447-8029

Elsevier Health Sciences Division
Subscription Customer Service
3251 Riverport Lane
Maryland Heights, MO 63043

*To ensure uninterrupted delivery of your subscription, please notify us at least 4 weeks in advance of move.

Printed and bound by CPI Group (UK) Ltd, Croydon, CR0 4YY

08/05/2025

01864717-0004